Language Signs and Calming Signals of Horses

Recognition and Application

Language Signs and Calming Signals of Horses

Recognition and Application

drs. Rachaël Draaisma
Behaviour Consultant and Trainer
Speaker – Author
Calming Signals of Horses
Milsbeek, The Netherlands

CRC Press
Taylor & Francis Group
Boca Raton London New York

CRC Press is an imprint of the
Taylor & Francis Group, an **informa** business

This book was translated from Dutch to English by Sarah Strous, Book Science Editing, Den Haag, The Netherlands.

CRC Press
Taylor & Francis Group
6000 Broken Sound Parkway NW, Suite 300
Boca Raton, FL 33487-2742

International Standard Book Number-13: 978-1-138-07015-8 (Hardback)

International Standard Book Number-13: 978-1-041-45073-3 (Paperback)

Library of Congress Cataloging-in-Publication Data

Names: Draaisma, Rachaël, author.
Title: Language signs and calming signals of horses : recognition and application / Rachaël Draaisma.
Description: Boca Raton : CRC Press, [2018]
Identifiers: LCCN 2017009168| ISBN 9781138070158 (hardback : alk. paper) | ISBN 9781138070158 (pbk. : alk. paper) |ISBN 9781315265667 (eBook)
Subjects: | MESH: Horses--psychology | Behavior, Animal
Classification: LCC SF281 | NLM SF 281 | DDC 636.1/0835--dc23
LC record available at https://lccn.loc.gov/2017009168

Visit the Taylor & Francis Web site at
http://www.taylorandfrancis.com

and the CRC Press Web site at
http://www.crcpress.com

For Product Safety Concerns and Information please contact our EU representative: GPSR@taylorandfrancis.com
Taylor & Francis Verlag GmbH, Kaufingerstraße 24, 80331 München, Germany

Contents

Foreword

Dear readers,

The moment you open this book and start reading it, you are taking part in an historic event. Twenty-five years ago, after years of study, I wrote the manuscript of my book about calming signals of dogs. I knew very well that all species share some of the same signals, and because I had worked with horses for a long time, I knew they also shared them. There was just never the time or the opportunity to undertake a study.

But I wished strongly that one day somebody would catch on to this idea and start studying horses and their language. One day I mentioned my dream to Rachaël, who was my dog trainer student at the time, and I glimpsed this fire light up her eyes – and I knew that this was the person to do it. And indeed she did! Studying, filming, photographing, recording more than I thought was possible, she ended up with an enormous amount of material to show people that horses do have calming signals, and that they do use them.

I am so happy to see this book become a reality; it is my dream come true as well as Rachaël's. Congratulations, Rachaël, I am so proud of you and your work, the result of your studies, and how it is manifested in the shape of this book. I hope all horse lovers and professionals will read it. Every person having anything to do with horses should; the importance of this book is unmeasurable.

In admiration of a fabulous piece of work,

Turid Rugaas
President of Pet Dog Trainers of Europe
Founder of TR International Dog Trainer Education
Owner of Hagan Hundeskole
Horse and Dog Behaviour Consultant and Trainer
Speaker – Author
Geithus, Norway

Introduction

'I don't understand why no one charts the calming signals of horses,' Turid Rugaas said during her International Dog Trainer Education course. I was her student, and her words stuck with me. By then I had already worked as a behavioural therapist for dogs for a number of years. Through the recognition and application of calming signals in dogs, my counselling of dogs and their owners had become highly specialised and refined. How incredible would it be, I thought, if this knowledge were also available to horse lovers. After all, like dogs, horses also face strict behavioural demands in our society. An additional tool would certainly be helpful here. Add to this my lifelong love of horses and the fact that I have owned a horse since the age of 14, and you can imagine that the idea of charting the calming signals of horses fascinated me. While setting up a resocialisation and man trailing programme for horses, I could not stop watching the signals they gave. It was not until a Sunday morning in 2013, however, that I decided to start this research and make a serious go of it. I was riding my horse in the woods and saw another rider approaching. The other horse wanted to have a look at my horse and so turned his head a little. He was immediately punished for this by his rider, who gave a forceful yank at the bit. A second attempt by the horse to turn his head slightly to look at us earned him a lash of the whip. The injustice of this moment made an impact on me. And although I might still not be able to prevent these kinds of situations in the future, I decided that I wanted to make a contribution to better communication between horses and people, in order to improve the welfare of horses. This has led to a major shift in my work. I had been working professionally with dogs and their owners since 2003. Now I rarely deal with dogs at all, and my week is filled with this research and working with horses.

GOAL OF THE RESEARCH

The goal of the research was to describe the calming signals of horses. These are the (relationship managing) signals that horses give in response to stimuli in their environment that they want to calm or appease in order to avert conflict and maintain social relationships – to be polite. Calming signals are also used when the horse wants to calm himself. However, to give a complete picture of the many ways in which a horse communicates and experiences the world, other communication signals were also added during the course of the research. These included calming signals, displacement activities, stress signals, and distance increasing signals.

It is important to me to describe the communication signals that a horse gives before tensions run so high that he becomes highly stressed or even runs or fights. In this state of maximum agitation, it is extremely difficult, if not impossible, to communicate with the horse. Instinctive reactions take over, and there is little or no room for cognitive reasoning and understanding. This brings with it serious health risks for rider and horse. Therefore, I wanted to chart the signals the horse gives before he reaches this high level of tension or shows severe fight or flight responses. There are many gradations that precede this and being able to recognise them is valuable. What does a horse look like when he is getting ever more tightly wound up? What does a horse look like when he wants to please a stimulus or stimuli in environment or wants to calm himself or another? If you recognise these signals, you can also deduce the stimuli your horse is responding to. You can assess the situation and make an informed decision. You can know if your horse can handle the situation or if you need to lend a hand by adjusting the circumstances a little. Recognising the communication signals of your horse better enables you to design a customised socialisation or training plan. It also improves your relationship with your horse, as well as his mental and physical health.

METHOD

I believed in an evidence-based approach to this research. I wanted my conclusions to be based on documentation, not on wishful thinking. That is why video footage forms the basis of the research. Alone and together with Ristin Olthof, I filmed domesticated horses in the Netherlands. Several people also sent me footage: videos of domesticated horses, mostly in the Netherlands but also a few from England and the United States. I categorised the videos and watched them repeatedly. I paid attention to the position of the ears, eyes, nose, mouth and tail of the horse. I also made note of the body postures and movements of horses and also people when they were present in the videos. I did not include vocal communications of the horse in this analysis.

I analysed 200 video recordings for this research. Every communication signal described in this book was seen at least 35 times to avoid overgeneralisation of a signal seen only once, so was possibly highly unusual. This means I might have assumptions about certain signals, but have not included them in this book because I have not yet seen them often enough or in sufficiently varied contexts to be confident about my view. The only exception to this can be found in Chapter 4 (section 4.3), which discusses learned helplessness. Just in that one instance, I report observations of my own that fell outside the scope of this research.

Footage was never staged or manipulated. If a person wanted to groom his horse, I asked if I could film it. The same was true for all sorts of situations: for example, when a horse was being saddled, brought to pasture, massaged, introduced to unfamiliar horses or people, or running free in the arena. This book is therefore based on real-life situations.

However, the term anecdotal evidence sometimes also applies. Communicative situations are unique. There can only be one first experience and only one first reaction to it. A horse brings the knowledge of that first time along to its second time, with the result that no two encounters can ever be called identical. 'Regrettably so,' I have sometimes thought, especially at times when I did not have my camera and, unforeseen, an interesting situation presented itself.

In one example, I saw a horse passing other horses and giving strong signals. When I had my camera ready the next day, eager to capture the same movements and facial expressions, the horse passed those same horses again without showing any of these signals. And why would he? He already knew them!

Also, I did not use any equipment to establish the heart rate, blood pressure or eye temperature of the horses studied in order to detect possible heightened tension.

THE HORSES

The research is based on domesticated horses. This is an important observation, as the behaviour of domesticated horses may differ greatly from that of horses living in the (semi) wild. This is due to their smaller environment, controlled living conditions, interaction with the world of humans, humans themselves, and the demands people make of domesticated horses. In this book, whenever I speak of horses, I mean domesticated horses and ponies who live in a domesticated world. Unless a horse is clearly identified as a female by her name, I use the masculine pronoun to refer to all the horses.

None of the horses filmed for this research had serious behavioural problems. As far as I knew, or could tell, they were all healthy. Nor does any of the material relate to horses who had visible physical injuries requiring veterinary attention. I also do not have video footage that shows behaviour or situations that led to extreme fight or flight responses. The videos are all of domesticated horses who, by human standards, are able to get along fine in our society. This does not mean they do not feel tension. These horses also experience mild to severe tension for short moments or longer periods. In addition, they communicate a lot, even if their handlers do not always know it.

When I started this research, I began to look at horses with a fresh eye. Not a single horse escaped this. Outside the planned moments for filming, I stopped by the side of the road whenever I saw horses. This might be when they were grazing at pasture, being led onto trailers, or being ridden by riders at home or in competitions. I wrote down my notes on scraps of paper or as text messages on my phone, or I recorded them as voice messages. Studying these horses was useful, but I did not have official consent from their owners to do so. Sometimes I did not even know who the owners were!

All the videos and photographs used in this book are included with the owners' consent. All the horses live in stables, where they have an individual stall in which they spend the night. They spend their days at pasture. The time they spend at pasture varies between 1 and 12 hours a day. Every horse is in contact with people on a daily basis. This is minimally twice a day, when they are taken to and collected from pasture, and maximally 10 times a day. This includes being taken and collected from pasture, being ridden, and being groomed. All the horses featured in this study are privately owned. None of the footage shows riding school horses. The age of the horses varies from 3 to 25 years old.

The breeds include Dutch and Belgian purebred horses, Friesians, Lipizzaners, Haflingers, New Forest ponies, Fjords, Tinkers, English Thoroughbreds, Quarter Horses, and Welsh Mountain ponies, as well as horses without pedigrees.

I am very aware that my study material focuses on horses who lead relatively good lives, with owners who allowed me and my camera into their world. Many horses live under bad conditions, horses whom I did not film, or whom I did film but whose owners did not give me permission to use the material.

CATEGORISATION AND COMMUNICATION LADDERS

My conclusions and choices are supported by video footage and analysis of this footage. As I scrutinised the footage, I began to discover signals that, as communicative signals, were new to me and that I had not read about as such in published works. These include several calming signals, such as looking away, blinking, half closing the eyes, showing the hindquarters, showing the flanks, and eating. I also noticed that certain behaviours kept coming back under certain circumstances.

Based on these groups of behaviours, I created communication ladders. These ladders each represent a situation and communication pattern that I observed during my research. They are schematic illustrations that, in a single glance, allow you to see how your horse's behaviour is related to stimuli in his everyday environment and whether his tension is building, or possibly decreasing, with the accompanying signals.

These communication ladders were then verified by first asking: does this safeguard the categorisation of behaviours? And second: is this categorisation and the explanation an easy tool to use for anyone who deals with horses? I categorised the behaviours as follows:

- Calming signals are behaviours that are aimed at appeasement, at avoiding conflict – being polite. Displaying these behaviours allows a horse to get through a situation while keeping social relations intact. Calming signals also enable any possible tension to discharge.
- Displacement activities too are behaviours that are meant to discharge tension. By focusing on something else and blocking out the circumstances around you, you can (sometimes according to learned social norms) get through a situation. But displacement activities involve physical behaviours that fall into a different behavioural group to the behaviours that occur before them.
- Stress signals are the signals a horse gives when the tension has risen to such a level that his body is preparing to take action by fight or flight.
- Distance increasing signals are the signals a horse will give when he is trying to stop a stimulus he finds disturbing or to put more distance between himself and the stimulus.

This study began as an investigation into calming signals only, but it turned out to require a number of additional dimensions. Of course it is possible for a horse to show only calming signals in a certain situation, but I have also seen many cases in which other signals flit through the calming signals, sometimes even taking over completely. Calming signals, displacement behaviours, stress signals, weakened fight or flight signals: the full range of body signals could, in a short time and in differing variations, be seen on film. Naming them all does more justice to reality and the varied way in which horses can react and communicate.

Sometimes my analyses of signals are new, sometimes they are the same as those made by other researchers, and sometimes they differ from them. For example, the categorisation of signals may differ. I categorise shaking of the neck as a calming signal. Other scientific researchers file it under displacement behaviour.

Hopefully my categorisations will bring recognition of the daily experiences you have with your horse, allowing you to better understand his behaviour in relation to the environment and enabling you to help him deal with it.

STRUCTURE OF THE BOOK

The book is organised as follows: Chapters 1 to 4 describe the different communication signals of horses. I also show what happens when the tension rises to a fight or flight response, as well as how the horse recovers from this. Chapter 1 addresses communication signals, stimuli and reactions. Chapter 2 covers calming signals and displacement activities. Chapter 3 tracks the process of rising tension until a fight or flight response occurs, followed by recovery. Chapter 4 deals with the situations in which horses no longer communicate at all, and Chapter 5 contains tips on how to use the calming signals to better understand your horse.

It is possible that as you read your horse's signals, you will start to view him and his behaviour in a different way. The information in this book can cause excitement and joy, but it can also cause feelings of uncertainty, spurring the sense that solutions must be found straight away. Nevertheless, I have chosen to bundle the tips in Chapter 5 and not disperse them in dribs and drabs in Chapters 1 to 4. This has allowed me to discuss the entire range of body signals and the information that goes with them step by step, without interruption, giving you, the reader, a broad and solid foundation for when you start reading the tips.

Every chapter follows the same structure. It starts with an introduction and a communication ladder that shows how a horse responds to a stimulus in his environment, including the associated signals. Then the communicative meaning of every individual body signal is discussed, accompanied by photographic material. Sometimes, for clarification or comparison, I discuss alternative functions of certain body signals or comparable communicative signals, allowing you to recognise your horse's behaviour even better. Every chapter ends with a summary.

Additionally, in the Appendix, for comparison purposes, there are several photos showing how horses use their eyes and ears.

HOW WILL THE BOOK HELP YOU?

This book is meant as a reference frame. It is full of photographs, enabling you to recognise your horse's behaviour. Learning to recognise your horse's behaviour is better than talking about it. The goal is for you to become better at reading your horse, more astute in spotting calming signals, displacement activities and stress signals, and better able to see which stimuli your horse can handle and which he cannot. Then the goal is for you to know what to do, and at an early stage too, before your horse's stress rises to such a level that it creates a negative climate in which to live, work and bond together. Because the book's overriding theme is calming signals, the tips in Chapter 5 are mostly focused on this, but also aim to make it as useful as possible. The tips are best applied to a horse who is relaxed or who feels slight tension. Such a horse is able to notice signals you give, think, reason, and remember. If, however, the two of you are in a situation that causes fear or pain in either you, the horse, or others, then consulting a veterinarian and a skilled behavioural therapist for horses is the best thing to do.

REFERENCES

Human beings, dogs, rats, horses. In science, these creatures are examined to gain a better understanding of human nature, and vice versa. Although there are obviously many differences between these species, there are also many similarities. For instance, humans and animals are very alike in how they physically respond to stress and how their brains work. The internet offers a wealth of sources that provide additional information about the different topics discussed in this book. In the References and Bibliography (personal favourites), I have listed some of the sources that are easily accessible, both in terms of purchase or perusal and of readability.

THE FUTURE

So does the publication of this book mean that I am done? Heavens no! This is only the beginning. I want to take a more detailed look at facial features. Several communication signals that I observed did not meet the inclusion criterion of 35 occurrences, but I will continue to study them as well as collect material. My large archive of videos and pictures of body signals keeps growing. This will allow me to better characterise these signals as well as others.

This study of the communication signals and calming signals of horses will continue for the rest of my life, so I can look forward to a future in which I will be able to decipher ever more communication signals.

I hope with all my heart that this book will help to make improve the lives of horses and lead to better communication between people and horses. Knowledge of this research has been so valuable to me in my contact with horses. I hope the same will be true for you.

Rachaël Draaisma

About the author

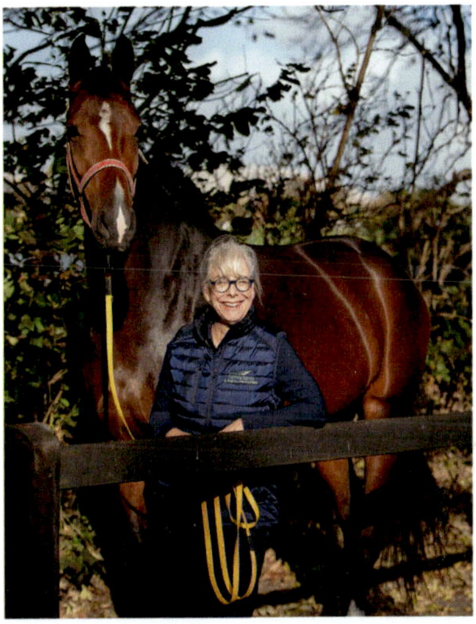

Rachaël graduated from Radboud University in Nijmegen, the Netherlands. She has always lived with and had a passion for dogs and horses, and in 2002 she decided to make it her profession. Rachaël achieved several diplomas and started working as a trainer and behavioural consultant, first with dogs and later with horses. In 2013 she completed the TR (Turid Rugaas) International Dog Trainers Education course. Under Turid's supervision she began studying how domesticated horses react to stimuli in their environment, including their 'calming signals' and how tension relates to these signals. The study led to the description of 20 calming signals that horses use to create and maintain a positive social climate and prevent negative escalation. It also led to the creation of communication ladders that show how horses may react to stimuli around them, a useful tool to assess the horse's tension and whether that tension is rising or declining. The study culminated in the worldwide publication of this book *Language Signs and Calming Signals of Horses*, an international bestseller translated into Chinese, Czech, Dutch, Polish and Finnish, with several other languages in preparation. Rachaël continues to study the communicative signals of horses, in particular their calming signals.

Another pillar of Rachaël's working life with horses evolves around equine mental stimulation and scentwork. Rachaël developed an extensive method to scent track with horses, in which she teaches horses to follow a footstep trail so they can find missing persons or scent bags. Tracking has enormous advantages for a horse's behaviour, brain, and body and it is also enriching for humans; scent work can therefore be seen as a new tool in enriching the human-equine relationship. Rachaël develops tracking to a level at which she uses it as a sole (primary) activity for horses. She also uses mental stimulation and scent tracking as a method when working with horses who have behavioural problems. Rachaël's second book *Scentwork for Horses* was published worldwide by CRC Press at the end of 2020.

To share her knowledge Rachaël travels throughout Europe and the globe to lecture about the calming signals of horses, equine mental stimulation and scentwork. She also gives workshops and a series of weekend sessions that combine theory and hands-on work with horses.

Acknowledgements

This research would not have got off the ground without Turid Rugaas, who inspired its inception and is a great mentor to me. Her philosophy and way of doing things shaped me as a trainer and behavioural therapist. Several tips and exercises from Chapter 5 were developed by Turid. For this, I am very grateful. Ristin Olthof is also one of the people who carried this project forward. She and I spent many hours filming and analysing footage together. Also, I could not have performed this research without the trust and help of the horse owners who gave me permission to film and those who sent me footage of their own. I am especially grateful to Anita Siks, Gertie Weijers, Jeanette Mäki, and the owners and boarding customers of Kösters Stables, 't Hof Stables, and B&B Angelbeeck. I am also very grateful to the test readers and motivators of the book: Marian Draaisma, Julia Robertson, Els Vidts, Anne LIll Kvam, Simon Jansen, Bert Peters (also my rock when it came to deciphering a number of computer programs), Robert Peters and Hans Ruijs. Many thanks to my friends and relatives who provided support, a well-moored and loving base, and of course, last but not least, my children Sybrand and Imke. They were supportive and patient with a mother who spent hours behind her computer and on the road to shoot footage. Not to mention one who talked about horses all the time. Not their cup of tea.

1 *The discovery of a language*

'The limit of my language means the limit of my world.' (Ludwig Wittgenstein)

BUTTERFLIES in my stomach, lots of energy, thoughts racing through my head. When I first started this research, it was as though I had fallen in love. I could think of nothing but this study and the signals horses give. I watched horses wherever and whenever I could. I filmed them and analysed footage.

I made note of body postures and movements and tried to find similarities. This seemed impossible during the first few months because I saw so many different signals. Also, at moments when I thought, 'Hey, it looks as though horses greet people by lowering their heads', I saw horses who did not do this. When I saw a horse who blinked his eyes when he felt tension, I also saw horses who did not blink but, for example, chewed.

During the first months I felt hopeful, confused, and sometimes a little desperate. But by tenaciously continuing to record and analyse footage, I began to see a much larger and more varied spectrum of signals that horses use. I now saw patterns I had not seen at the beginning, because my field of vision had been too narrow. I needed to see and recognise more signals in order to place them inside a broader spectrum.

During my study I looked at the signals horses use in their domesticated living environment. How a horse understands and experiences his living conditions, how he responds to stimuli, and how much he communicates depends on a number of factors:

- The genetic disposition he has inherited from his ancestors; his physiology, the way in which his brain and organs work; his endocrine system; and whether he has inherited a susceptibility to any diseases or a sensitivity to fear and stress; his anatomical structure and biomechanical functions.
- His health. He may be incidentally stressed, chronically stressed, or depressed. He may be in pain. He may also feel especially relaxed, because all his mental and physical needs are being met.
- His experiences in life, both positive and negative, which to a greater or lesser degree enable him to deal flexibly with his life.
- His socialisation and training, which can either be a positive or a negative contribution to the horse's ability to cope with his life.
- His rider or handler, on whom the domesticated horse is highly dependent. A domesticated horse's quality of life is closely related to the choices made by his owner or handler.

- His living environment, which has to meet the horse's needs. Is there enough room to move? Shelter? Is there enough for him to eat and drink? Is there an opportunity for social contact with other horses? Can he get enough rest and sleep? Is he able to make choices? Does he have the option of withdrawing from certain stimuli he finds difficult to handle, or is he forced to undergo these stimuli because of a lack of space or freedom of choice?

NO TWO HORSES ARE THE SAME

There are so many possible combinations of the above points that I am confident in saying that no two horses are the same, live the same life, get treated the same way, or experience the world in the same way. There are always differences in genetics, how the horse is housed, or the way his rider or handler treats him. Then there are variations in breeding and foaling programmes, socialisation, training, reward, punishment, contact with other horses, contact with people or other animals, the degree to which the horse is free to make choices, the number of times the horse is sold or moved, and generally differences in associations with all sorts of stimuli in the environment. Getting to know your horse is one of the most wonderful things to undertake. Finding out what he can and cannot handle, what he likes, and what he finds easy and difficult enables you to know if you should help him through a situation or step back. Getting to know your horse will strengthen your bond. It will also allow you to optimally guide your horse in every facet of his life, whether it is focused on dressage, show jumping, walking, recreational riding, Western riding, or ordinary daily living.

1.1 COMMUNICATION SIGNAL OR NOT?

A sigh while walking, a whinny when greeting, scraping the floor with a foreleg while begging for a treat: most owners know their horse's habits. Although horses also communicate vocally, in this book I look only at their body language, especially the body signals and language related to responding and communicating.

But of course, the question is, when is a horse using his body to respond and communicate and when is he not? After all, a horse also uses his body to execute natural behaviours related to eating, drinking, resting, and procreating. The horse yawns when he is tired, half closes his eyes when he is falling asleep, scrapes his hoof across the floor to toss up ground and smell, and shakes sand from his body when he has been rolling. Here are a few pointers to help you start characterising your horse's body signals:

- Body signals and/or communication signals are always situation specific.
- The entire situation has to be taken into consideration. What is happening? What is not happening? And what is the horse responding to? It is like watching a scene in a play. What is the setting? Who are the characters? And what is the storyline?
- Paying attention to the context is crucial. Imagine your horse is at pasture and a bumble bee flies at his head. He shakes his head at the bumble bee. In this situation, his head shaking is related to chasing off the bumble bee.
- Imagine you are walking your horse around the arena. Parallel to the arena is a public road, and on it a tractor is noisily making its way in your direction. When the tractor passes you, your horse stops to take a look at it. As he watches the tractor pass by, your horse chews and blinks his eyes. He moves his head down and back up once and starts walking. The initial stimulus for his body signals is the tractor, and the horse may be responding to the tractor's appearance, its sound, its passing by or its driving away, a combination of these options, or all of these options.
- It is self-evident that in stimulus-rich environments there are many stimuli to which your horse may be responding, and you will have to figure out whether he is reacting to all the stimuli, to one of them, or to a number of them.

HORSES ALSO RESPOND TO AND COMMUNICATE WITH OBJECTS AND VISUAL AND AUDITORY STIMULI

People often think that communication is only possible between humans and animals, or between animals and other animals. However, the communication patterns I have seen horses display towards people and other animals, I have also seen them display towards inanimate objects. These might be items such as rocks or trash bins, visual stimuli such as shadows or flickers of light, or sounds such as a cow mooing in the distance, the tinkling of a dreamcatcher, or a leaf blower.

CERTAIN GROUPS OF SIGNALS BELONG TOGETHER

This means that there are different signals within the group of calming signals, different signals in the group displacement activities, etc. Within each group of communication signals, every horse uses its own particular signals. Horses seem to have personal preferences and form habits. In meeting a dog, for example, one horse might wish to avoid trouble and be polite, showing calming signals by chewing or tongue out chewing, or doing both. Another horse might turn his head away. Yet another might do a combination of the two, and maybe blink his eyes as well. Certain groups of signals keep coming back in all horses at the same moments.

THE COMMUNICATION SIGNALS REFLECT THE INTERNAL CONDITION OF THE HORSE

Horses do not lie. Their posture and body language show how they feel and what their intentions are. Are you seeing stress signals? Then the horse is stressed. Are you seeing distance increasing signals? Then the horse wants to create more space between himself and others. Emotions and signals come and go according to how the horse is feeling.

How a horse experiences a stimulus, how he responds and communicates, can be deduced from his body signals. These are different depending on the situation. If a horse is feeling a little awkward about the sound of a lawnmower, he may show one calming signal. If the same horse is very awkward about the sound of a tractor, then he may show five calming signals.

After a while, a horse may, through personal growth and experience, come to show different signals in identical situations, so after a period of socialisation he might no longer show any calming signals at all. For me, therefore, it is crucial to keep watching and to support your claims with evidence. Just saying, 'And then the horse got angry', without backing this up by pointing to body signals the horse is showing at the time, is an admission of weakness. It is making assumptions. If you think your horse is angry, but when you look at him you see only stress signals and attempts to leave the situation, you have to change your assessment.

THERE IS INTERACTION

If your horse is showing signals and you or others in the vicinity are responding to them, then a new situation has arisen. There is action and reaction. Communication and interaction are taking place. On both sides, signals are adapted to the other or to the situation.

1.2 IT ALL STARTS WITH A STIMULUS AND A REACTION

A horse who startles and jumps sideways shows behaviour that we always recognise and respond to. However, horses also have body signals and facial expressions that are less obvious, sometimes smaller and quieter. Many riders and handlers do not see them or do not attach meaning to them. Some riders and handlers do recognise them, but do not know what an appropriate response might be. This is a missed opportunity. After all, you want to guide your horse in such a way that high tension and fight or flight responses are avoided. In terms of communication, this requires two things: (1) you have to recognise the body signals of your horse, and (2) you have to recognise the initial stimulus (i.e. the stimulus that causes communicative behaviour or a pattern of behaviours).

It might be a challenge to identify the initial stimulus to which your horse is responding. You may have been lost in thought, not paying attention to your horse's environment. It might also be that your horse's environment is so familiar to you that you cannot imagine your horse responding at all. It might even be the case that your horse is responding to a visual, auditory, or sensorimotor stimulus that you cannot perceive because human senses evolved differently.

People often respond with the help of a kind of helicopter view. They rise above a situation and analyse it as the result of a larger whole. If, for example, a horse has a startle response, they may say it is because: 'My horse has not been properly socialised', or 'He is young', or 'He is always easily spooked when it is windy out'. And yes, of course, the fact that your horse is young or not well socialised contributes to his startle response. It can also certainly be a cause of it. But I want you to start distinguishing between a cause and a trigger. The trigger is the initial stimulus that causes the horse to display certain behaviour. You will find the trigger, or the initial stimulus, by asking yourself what happened the moment before your horse started? Did a bird fly out of the bushes? Was there a sound? A shadow? Stop and listen. Look around you. Was it one stimulus or were there more than one? Watch your horse. What is he looking at? Knowing which stimuli trigger your horse is necessary in order to help him, and to make a plan to enable him to deal with his environment.

2 *Calming signals to appease and calm*

2.1 WHAT ARE CALMING SIGNALS?

It is a warm, sunny day. You are sitting at a pavement café with a friend, chatting. You take a sip of tea and lean back in your comfortable chair. You watch people passing by, a whole range of shapes and colours. A woman with red curls briskly marching by, a child skipping, a sturdy dame with a little dog, and an older man with a slight limp. Your eye lingers on the man. You watch him approach the café. He stops in front of it, his gaze roaming the tables. At your table, his eyes pause. He looks you straight in the eye, his expression open. For a second, you do not know what to do. Say hello? Nod? Stare back? You answer his stare with a friendly smile and a nod. The man looks away and resumes his slow walk down the street. You take another sip of your tea, wondering why the man had been staring at you.

This scenario shows how a situation in which there is no communication between the person at the café and the passers-by changes into a situation in which communication between the limping man and the person drinking tea is initiated. This communication can feel very natural, in which case you give a signal, a nod or a smile, almost without conscious thought. It can also feel like a purposeful action, such as when, in my case, I say, 'Hello' when entering a hotel elevator crammed with silent, staring people.

The purpose of offering these types of responses is to calm and appease the other person or people in order to achieve or maintain a positive living environment, protect any social relationships, and prevent negative escalations. Just like humans, dogs, and undoubtedly many other mammals, horses also use these calming signals. It is not surprising that horses have developed these communicative skills, specifically. Horses naturally live in groups. Good, stable friendships and familial relations ensure safety, a good life, and survival. Also, preventing conflicts and their attendant injuries or forced isolation is of great importance to horses. Just like dogs and humans, horses are able to form relationships outside their own species, and they use the same signals to communicate with these other species that they use with other horses.

In addition to calming people, animals, and other environmental stimuli, calming signals have one other important function: they reduce the horse's own tension. Of course, the difference between when the horse is calming itself and when he is trying to calm others can be difficult to spot. Personally I work under the assumption that when a horse is trying to appease a person, when he is managing a social relationship, he communicates with that person. On film, you will see the horse give one or two calming signals, look at the person or other stimulus he is communicating with for a reaction, and possibly give another calming signal. So there are pauses between calming signals during which the horse checks for possible responses.

When the horse is calming himself, however, you will often see him give calming signals without making direct contact with his environment. In my opinion, calming signals fulfil both functions at the same time: the horse calms both himself and other stimuli.

Within the group of calming signals, I will name the 20 that are most common. That does not mean that your horse will show every one of these signals in order, or even use all of them. Horses vary when it comes to calming signals, and they also seem to develop personal habits in their use of them.

Where one horse may blink a lot to calm himself and others, another may chew more. One horse will show a sequence of blinking, looking away, and chewing, another will sooner shake his neck and turn away. Every horse has his own time frame in which he is able to deal with a situation.

As a general rule:

1 When a horse uses calming signals, he can use one or more of them.
2 When a horse shows multiple signals, they can follow one another.
3 It is also possible, however, for two or three signals in a sequence to be given simultaneously.

DOES A HORSE FEEL TENSION IF HE SHOWS A CALMING SIGNAL?

In this research, I did not use any equipment to measure eyeball temperature, heart rate, or blood pressure, or do a saliva or blood test to measure stress and hormone levels. My answer to this question, therefore, is based on analysing video footage. I see horses giving calming signals when they:

1 Have a relaxed posture and a relaxed facial expression. Calming signals meant to appease people, animals, or other stimuli in the environment are normal communication tools of horses. They are given in everyday circumstances to maintain social relationships. Other than in the very brief moment before the horse gives the calming signal, they do not produce added tension. Therefore, the horse is relaxed, there is a stimulus, the horse registers this in a moment of light tension, gives a calming signal, and then relaxes again. This includes, for instance, when one or two calming signals are given, possibly with a pause in between signals while the horse checks for a response.
2 Experience tension, but the tension either stays level or increases. Here the horse gives calming signals during or right after the stimulus or situation that is causing his tension. But the tension does not go away. Instead of relaxing after having given the calming signal, the horse stays tense for a time or the tension even increases.

3 Experience tension, but the severe tension is decreasing. The horse was very tense, but the stimulus or situation that caused it has stopped. The horse is recovering from the higher tension. On the descent into relaxation, when the tension is decreasing, he gives calming signals.

THE MORE CALMING SIGNALS THERE ARE, THE HIGHER THE TENSION

If I take a bird's eye view of calming signals, I can see that the more calming signals a horse gives in a short time, and the faster they succeed one another, the sooner the horse will show displacement behaviour (see section 2.24), stress signals (see section 3.2), or both. If a horse shows multiple calming signals simultaneously or sequentially in a single moment, in my opinion he is definitely experiencing tension or rising tension.

If the horse experiences elevated tension and then this tension drops, you will see that the horse, when he has calmed down enough to use calming signals, often initially uses see-saw lowering (see section 2.15) when he is still moving. Then when he briefly stops (coming from a walk, trot, or canter) he gives a neck shake (see section 2.13) or body shake (see section 2.14). He does not start to use the smaller signals such as blinking and chewing until there is more relaxation and less physical activity.

A horse shows a pendular pattern when he displays ambivalent behaviour, when multiple behaviour systems are active consecutively or simultaneously, and the horse feels contradictory motivations. This is discussed in more detail in Chapter 5.

It is important to be able to discern whether your horse's tension is increasing or decreasing.

When your horse starts giving calming signals, there is no tension or only light tension. The horse can remain in his current state if you think he is able to recover and relax (with or without your help), and then actually does so! The moment a horse gives stress signals, his body is preparing to either flee from the situation or fight it. Whether this actually happens depends on the guidance the horse receives and on the handler's ability to adapt the situation in such a way that the horse is able to cope with it. In order to make a good assessment of your horse, it helps to:

1 Read body signals, such as calming signals, displacement behaviour, stress signals, and distance increasing signals.
2 Analyse the face and body posture of your horse.

It is Sunday morning. I am standing on a path, next to some paddocks, looking at Prince. The paddock is next to a public road. He is grazing. A car passes. Prince looks up. He holds his head mid-high and his ears are pointed forward, towards the car. His eyes are almond-shaped and his nostrils long. His mouth is not clenched. His lower lip slightly protrudes in front of his upper lip. His tail hangs down, a relaxed position. After a few seconds he returns to his grazing, flank facing the road. A few minutes later, a cyclist passes by. I see Prince's left ear move. It follows the cyclist. But he does not look up, and keeps grazing. Some minutes pass, and then Prince raises his head high. His eyes are round. His mouth is closed, but not clenched. His nostrils move from long to round and back again. A man in an electric wheelchair passes by. Prince does not move, and stays motionless for a good 8 seconds. Then he blinks and chews. The man in the electric wheelchair is out of sight, but can still be heard. After a few seconds, Prince returns to his grazing.

In this scenario, Prince hardly has any trouble with the car or the cyclist, or he is not interested in them and does not initiate communication. However, the electric wheelchair prompts him to respond. He gives three calming signals, and his face also reflects light tension.

When my horse is attended by a farrier, he shows no calming signals when three of his hooves are trimmed. However, when the farrier gets to his left hind leg, on lifting the leg my horse starts to show calming signals, such as tongue out chewing. When the farrier is finished, the horse no longer gives any signals. To me, this is a sign that the horse has trouble lifting this particular leg. It could be that it causes him physical pain or that he feels some lingering negative associations from the past, for example, because thrush (a common infection of the hoof) was scraped out once, and this hurt.

But keep paying close attention to the entire situation and context. What if the horse starts chewing when the farrier lifts his left hind leg, but at the same time someone walks into the stable? The horse's calming signal could also have been for the person. It helps to know which stimulus your horse saw, heard, or felt before or during the calming signal.

As discussed in Chapter 1, a horse's body movements can have different functions. By analysing the context of your horse's movements, you can bring clarity to this. The communication ladder below shows the lines of communication and calming signals that apply when a horse gives calming signals in response to a new stimulus.

2.2 COMMUNICATION LADDER: CALMING SIGNALS

Ladder 2.1

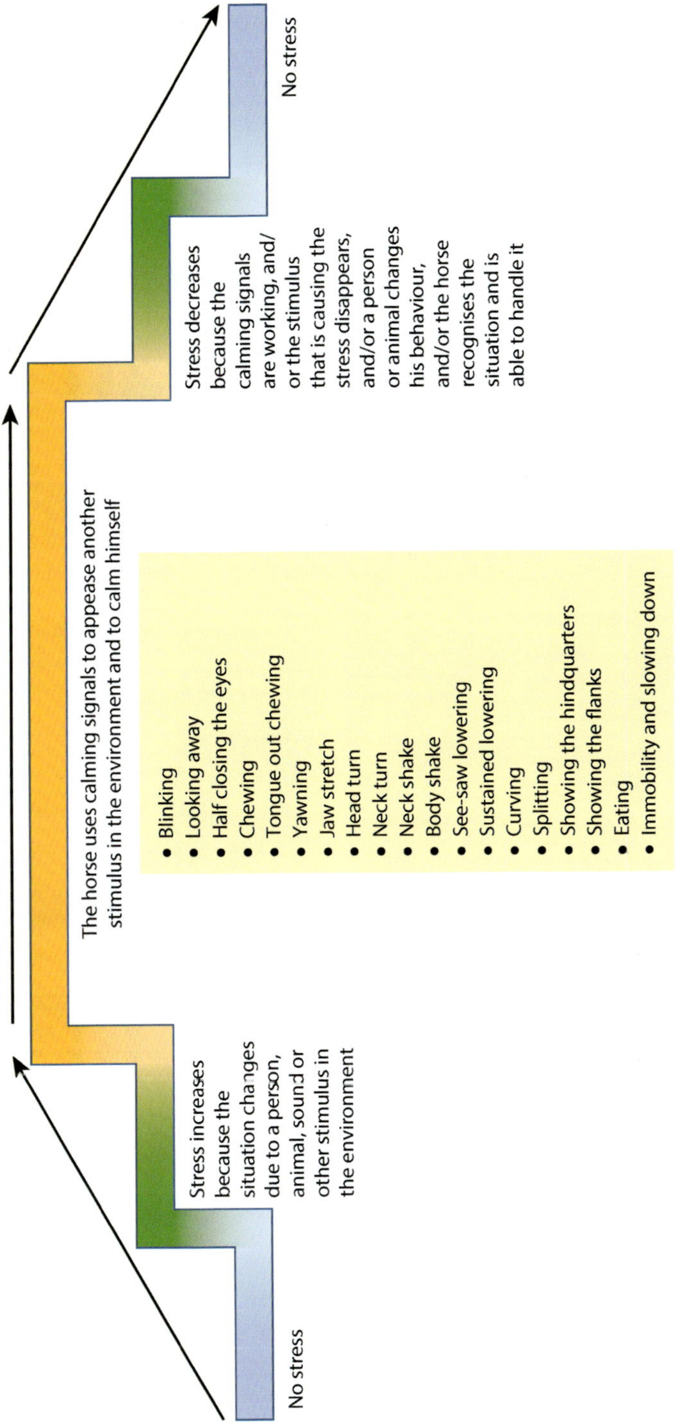

2.3 BODY POSTURE

Calming signals can be seen in all possible head–neck positions: low, mid-low, horizontal, mid-high, and high (**Figs 2.1–2.6**). However, most calming signals are seen in the mid-high and horizontal positions. Any position of the ear is possible: for example, both ears forward, sideways, turned back, one ear forward and one sideways. Should signals have any special features, this will be explained alongside the signal in question.

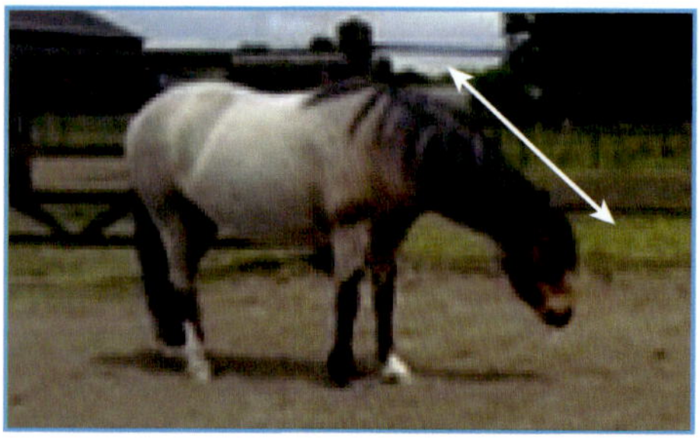

Fig. 2.1 The lowest head–neck position.

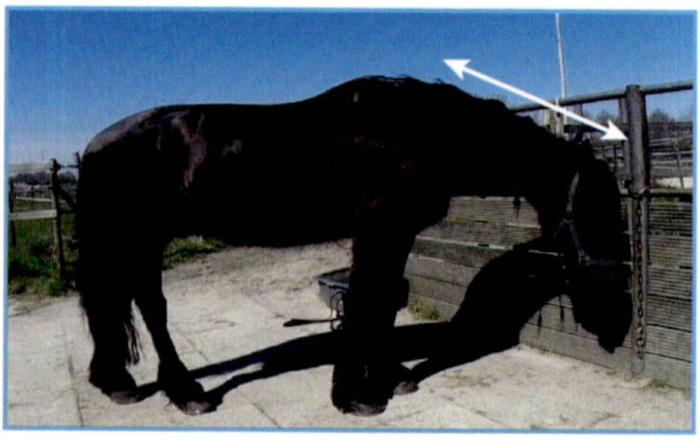

Fig. 2.2 A mid-low head–neck position.

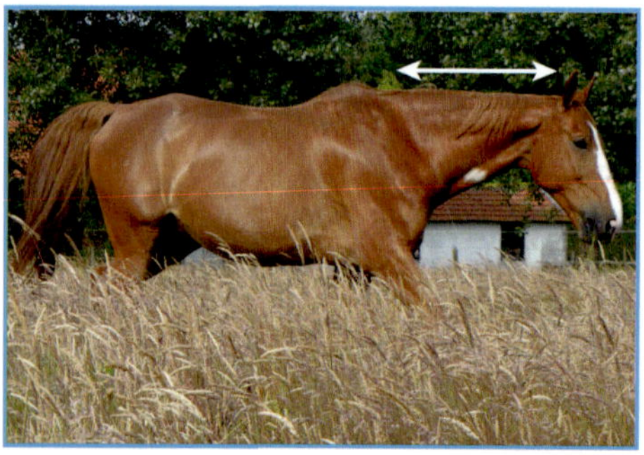

Fig. 2.3 A horizontal head–neck position.

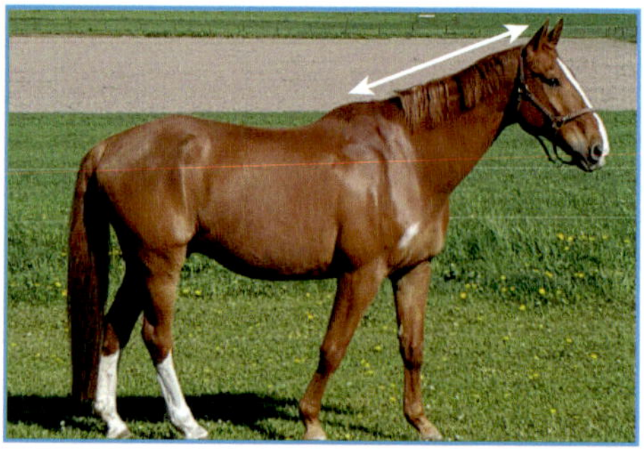

Fig. 2.4 A mid-high head–neck position.

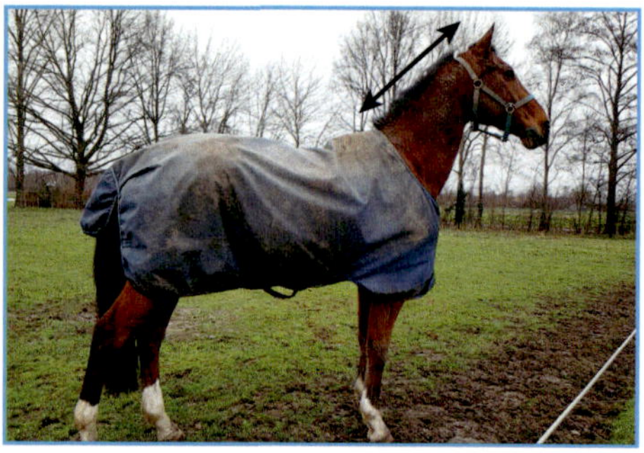

Fig. 2.5 The highest head–neck position.

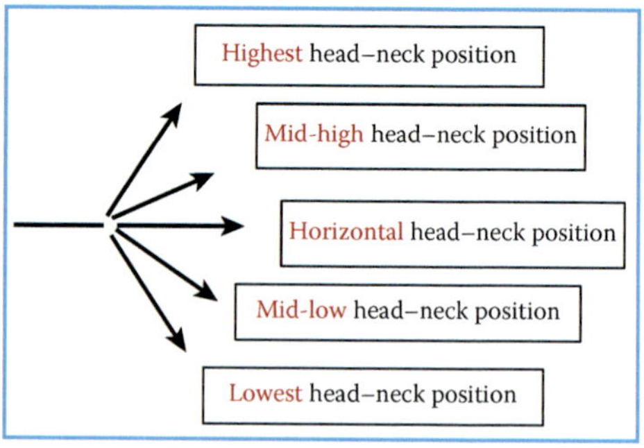

Fig. 2.6 Schematic diagram of the head–neck positions.

2.4 FACIAL FEATURES AND TAIL CARRIAGE

Calming signals are given both when the horse is relaxed and when he experiences tension. To judge this, look at your horse's face and the way he carries his tail. Described below is how you will see these elements in cases of relaxation.

WHEN THE HORSE IS RELAXED

***A relaxed face is smooth, without wrinkles* (Figs 2.7–2.10)**

The horse's face looks smooth. There are no wrinkles between the nostrils and the mouth. The jaws are not clamped together, so there is no tight line or thickening of the area that extends beyond the seam of the mouth. The chin is not pronounced and it extends in a fairly straight line to the cheek.

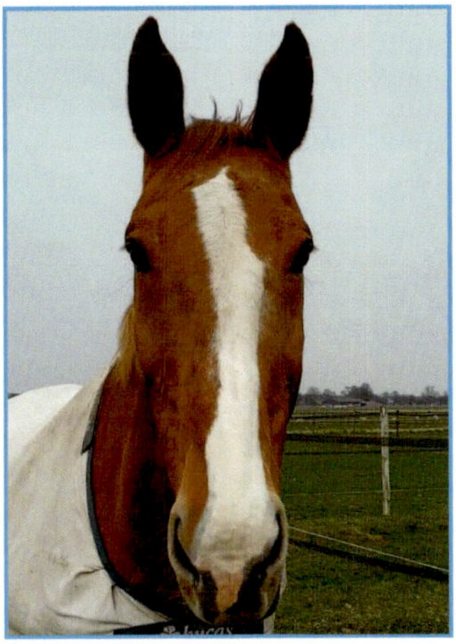

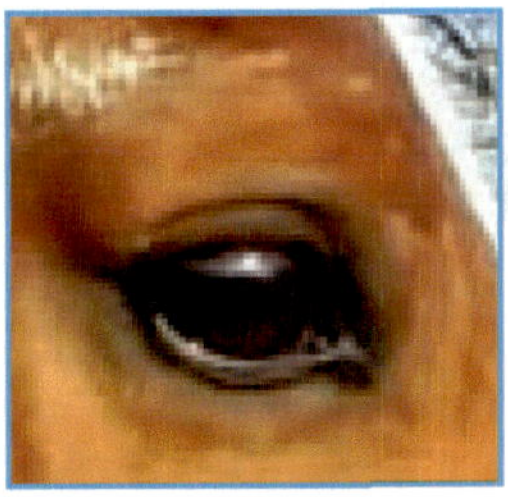

Figs 2.7, 2.9 Relaxed eyes are almond-shaped.

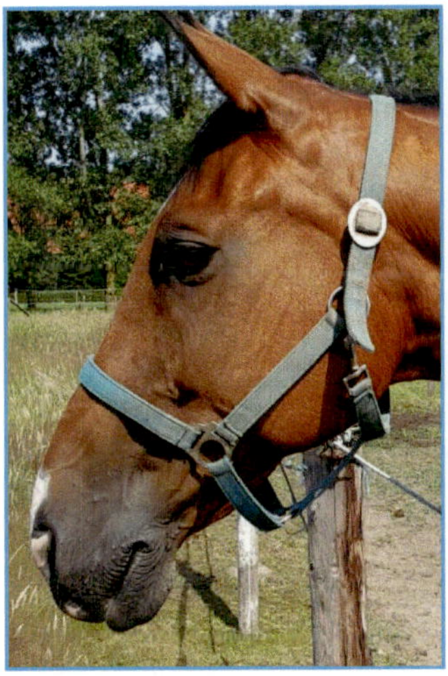

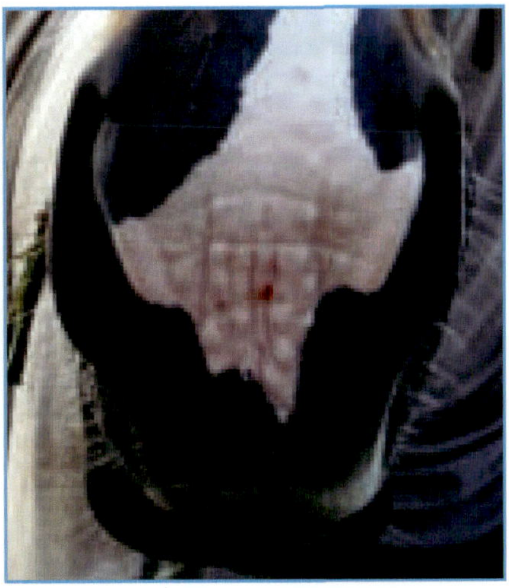

Figs 2.8, 2.10 Relaxed nostrils are long.

***A relaxed mouth has soft, closed lips* (Figs 2.11, 2.12)**

It is also possible that the rim of the lower lip or a corner of the lower lip is visible or that the lower lip protrudes slightly in front of the upper lip.

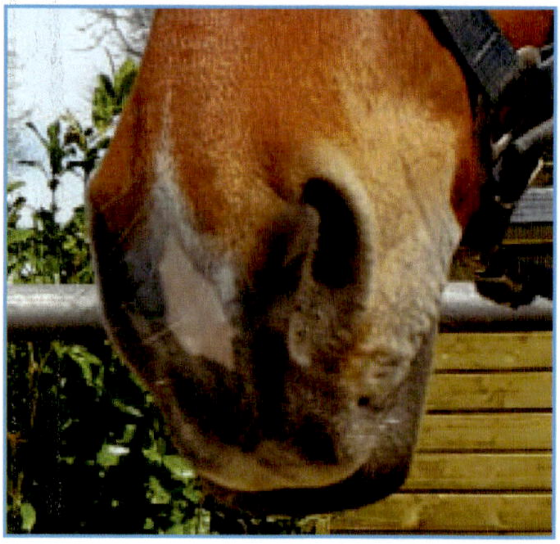

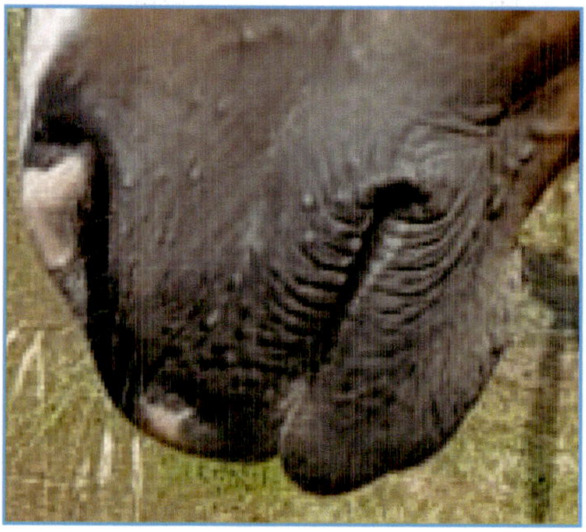

Figs 2.11, 2.12 A relaxed mouth with soft, closed lips.

NOTE: A lower lip that is slightly longer than the upper lip is also a body feature of older horses, so even when these horses experience tension, the lower lip may still protrude in front of the upper lip.

***A relaxed chin is not tensed* (Fig. 2.13)**

A relaxed chin feels soft and connects to the lower jaw in a straight line.

***A relaxed tail hangs calmly and loosely* (Fig. 2.14)**

The tail hangs down in a relaxed fashion, so the base of its tail is not tense.

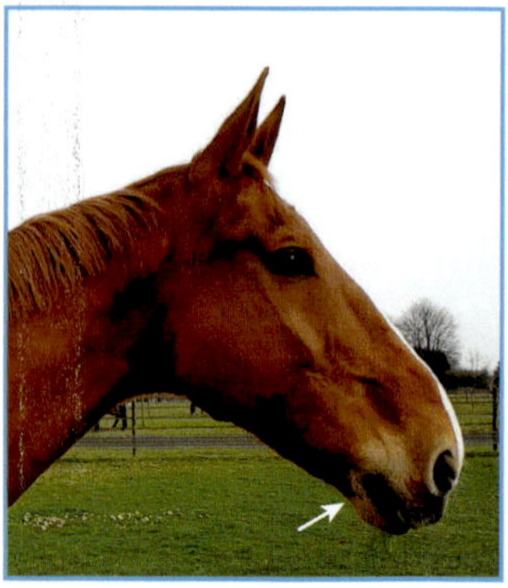

Fig. 2.13 Relaxed chin (arrow).

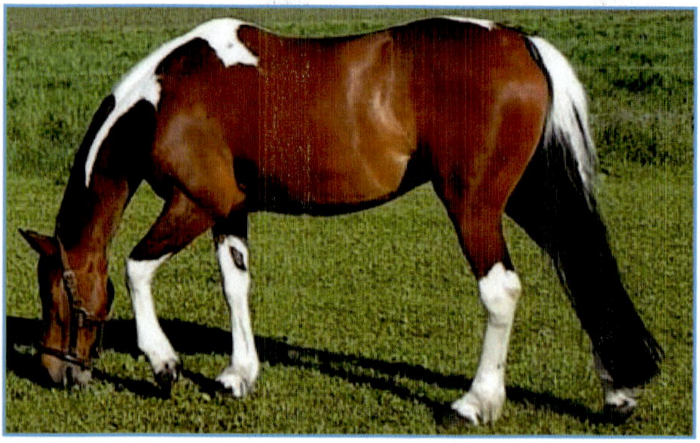

Fig. 2.14 Tail hanging down in a relaxed fashion.

WHEN THERE IS LIGHT TENSION

When you look at the eyes, mouth, and nose of a horse, you will see that when he feels light tension his mouth is still relaxed, as described in the previous paragraph. However, the eyes or nostrils, or both, are round and tense. The nostrils may go from long to round and back again as the horse smells and breathes more heavily. You might see light tension when a horse is investigating a stimulus by smell and/or sight or is in a situation that causes him light tension. The photos below show some variations that can occur (**Figs 2.15–2.17**).

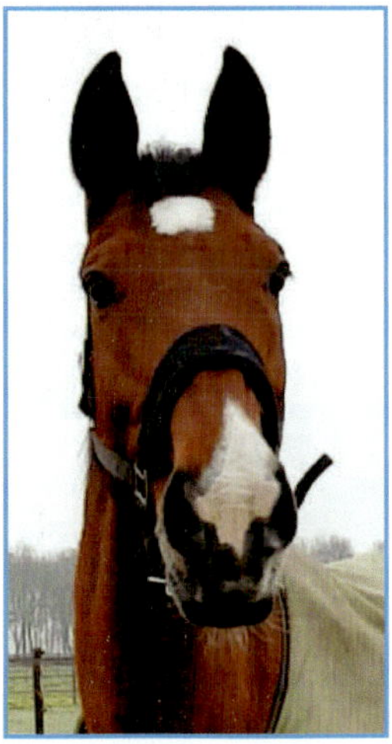

Fig. 2.15 Nostrils: tense and rounder due to an active olfactory sense. Eyes: relaxed and almond-shaped. Mouth: relaxed.

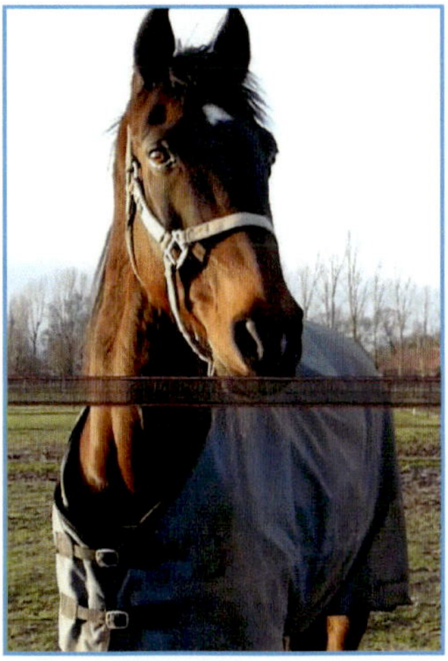

Fig. 2.16 Eyes: tense and round due to more active watching behaviour. Nostrils: relaxed and long. Mouth: relaxed.

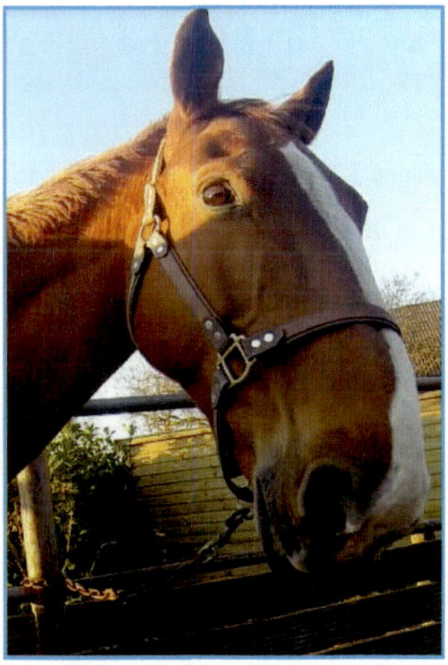

Fig. 2.17 Eyes: tense and round. Nostrils: tense and round. Mouth: relaxed.

The tail

The tail of a horse who notices a stimulus or experiences a situation with light tension hangs down in a relaxed fashion or is carried lightly (**Figs 2.18, 2.19**).

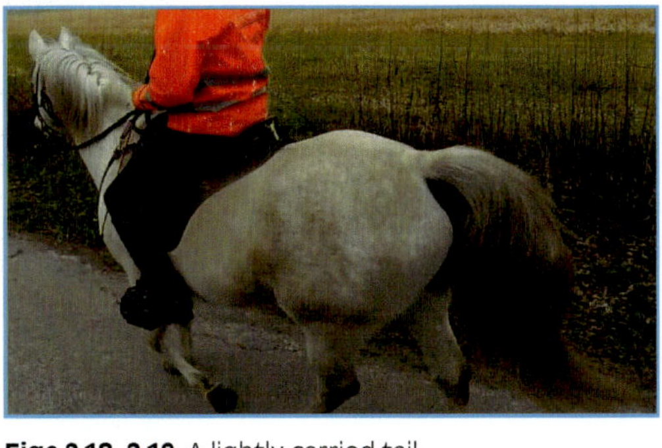

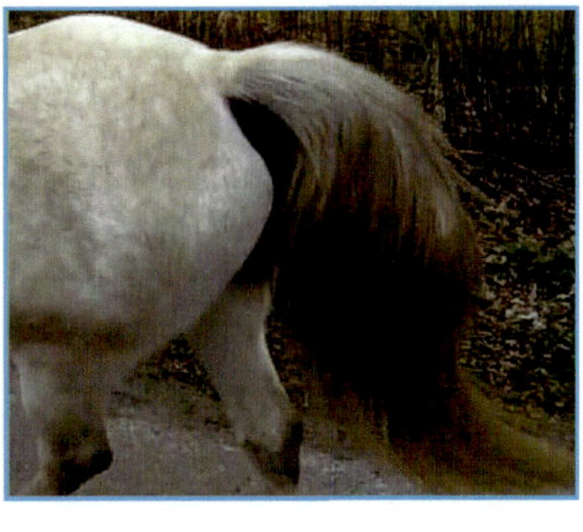

Figs 2.18, 2.19 A lightly carried tail.

2.5 BLINKING

Blinking is one of the smallest calming signals. If you are not paying attention when a horse blinks, you will miss it. However, you will often get a second chance. After a pause of a few seconds, the horse often repeats the blinking. It can also be part of a pattern: blink-blink-blink – pause of a few seconds – blink-blink-blink. Most horses who use blinking as a calming signal are standing still or walking when they do so. Blinking the eyes is often the first calming signal.

*Lectron is at pasture. I walk towards him, filming him. He watches me (**Fig. 2.20**) and blinks at me as a calming signal (**Fig. 2.21**). Then he watches me for a response (**Fig. 2.22**). The blinking is an appeasement signal for me and also functions as a calming signal for himself. Lectron feels light tension. His eyes are round, his nostrils are long, and his tail is relaxed (not visible).*

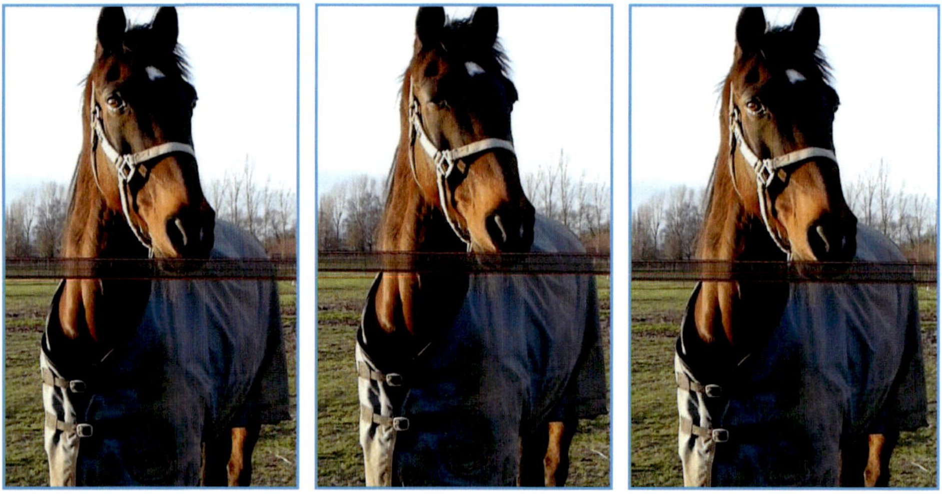

Figs 2.20–2.22 Blinking.

Blinking occurring at the same time as another calming signal, the neck turn (see section 2.12), is shown (**Figs 2.23–2.28**). Blinking can also occur as a protective response (**Fig. 2.29**).

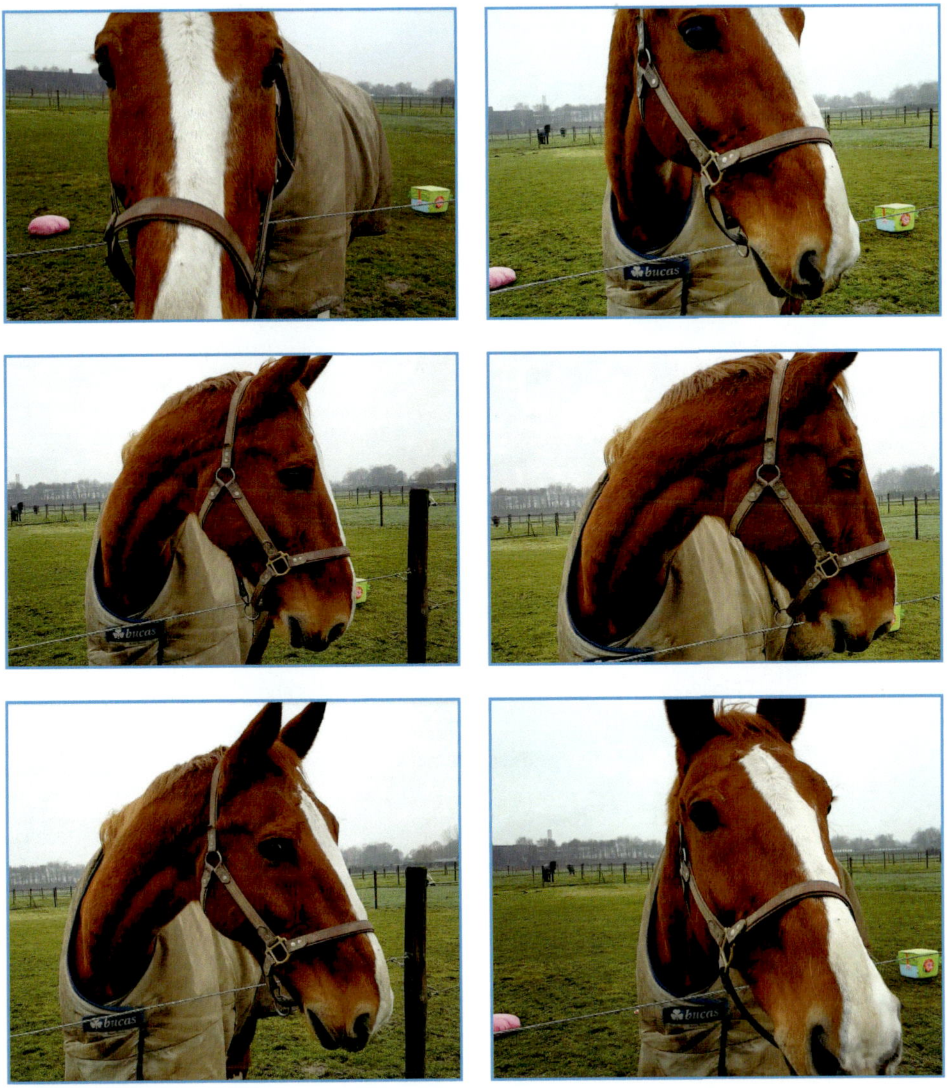

Figs 2.23–2.28 ***Top left:*** Vosje looks at me with both eyes (binocular) as I film him. I do not respond and keep filming. ***Top right:*** Vosje looks at me with one eye (monocular). ***Middle left:*** Vosje looks away with his eyes and begins a neck turn (see section 2.12) as a calming signal. ***Middle right:*** Vosje blinks his eyes (calming signal) while, as a calming signal, he also makes a neck turn (see section 2.12). ***Bottom left:*** Vosje turns back to me. His upper lip extends forward slightly to… ***Bottom right:*** rub it over my arm.

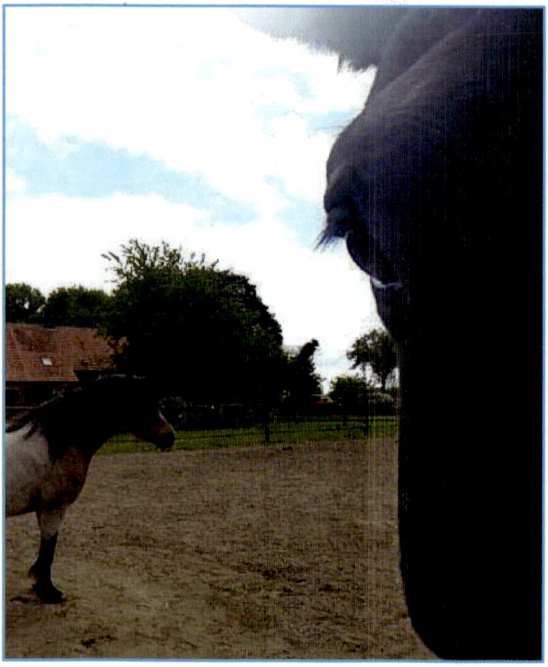

Fig. 2.29 Blinking as a response to the fly that is about to land near the eye. The blinking has no communicative meaning here; it is for the protection of the eye.

2.6 HALF CLOSING THE EYES

Half closing the eyes is a calming signal where the amount of time during which the eye remains half closed is the variable. Half closing the eyes may be a brief instance within a communication sequence of calming signals. For example, you will see a horse blink his eyes, close them for half a second, and then look away. Or the horse may half close his eyes for a longer time. It appears as though the horse is taking a break during the communication without wanting to provoke the other horse or person. Half closing the eyes can last for 2–10 seconds, until another communicative signal or action happens.

Some girls are waiting on a bike path. They are standing at the edge of a paddock, slouching over their bikes. One girl turns towards a horse. She watches him, her body fully facing him. The horse holds his head mid-high. He blinks his eyes and looks away, then half closes his eyes. The girl keeps watching. After 4 seconds, the horse turns and walks away.

Half closing the eyes to avoid conflict also applies when horses are standing very close to one another or to people and there is very little physical room to give other signals (**Fig. 2.30**).

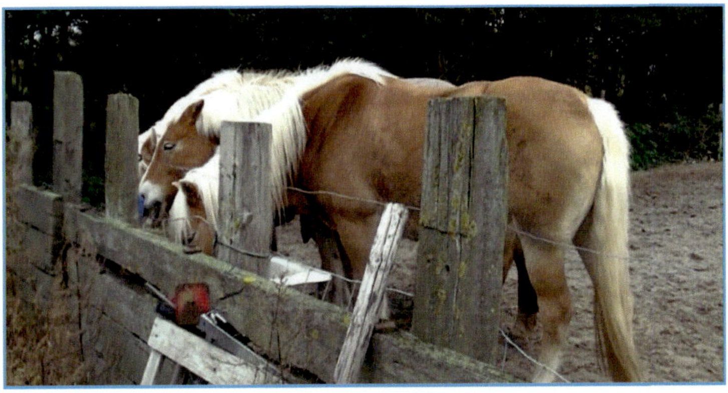

Fig. 2.30 Haflingers eating from the same hay trough. At the start of the meal, when they are positioning themselves, there is always some commotion over who stands where. Now they are all gathered in close to eat. The horse in the middle eats with her eyes half closed so does not incite conflict.

Half closing the eyes has another function, namely as protection, for example, when a halter or bridle is being put on or against outside forces such as insects, hail, or snow. You also see half closed eyes in horses who are 'nodding off' and falling asleep. Other features in this horse are that the ears are turned sideways and there is a head–neck position that is somewhere between mid-high and mid-low. The tail is hanging down in a relaxed fashion.

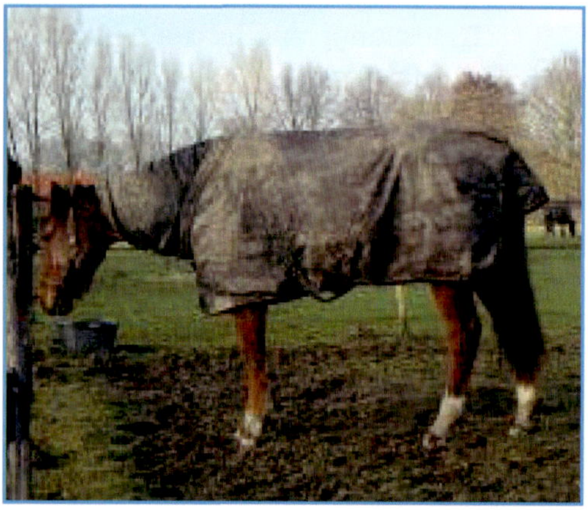

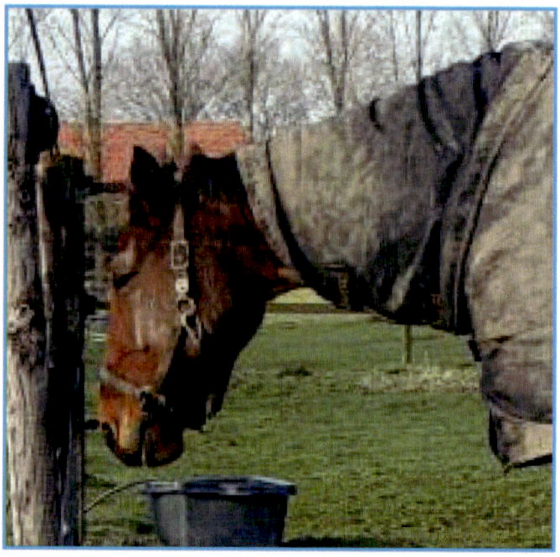

Figs 2.31, 2.32 A horse who is 'nodding off'.

Half closing the eyes, together with a horizontal or mid-low head–neck position, is also something you see in horses who are in pain, depressed or have descended into a learned mode of helplessness, closing themselves off from stimuli around them. This is discussed in more detail in Chapter 4.

2.7 LOOKING AWAY

When I was 24, I hosted three elderly Australian ladies as house guests. They were Aboriginals, and the oldest had spent the first years of her life in a small community of Aborigines, where she had been raised according to the values of her people. When she got to primary school, she received angry reactions from her Australian teachers because she would not look them in the eye when they were talking. To the Australian teachers, this was a sign of disrespect. My guest, however, had been taught differently. In her culture it was a sign of respect not to look an elder in the eye. After all, the eyes are the mirrors to the soul. Not just anyone is allowed to look into them.

Looking away as a calming signal is something a horse will mostly do when he is standing still. When he looks away as a calming signal, he breaks off his view of a stimulus. He hardly changes position as he does it, although a small movement of the head, a few centimetres to the left or right, away from the stimulus, is also possible.

There are two ways in which a horse can look away:

1 He can do so by no longer directing his gaze outward to see, but turning it more inward. The eye also seems to become duller when this happens.
2 He can change his viewing direction.

The photos (**Figs 2.33–2.36**) show an example of looking away by turning the gaze more inward.

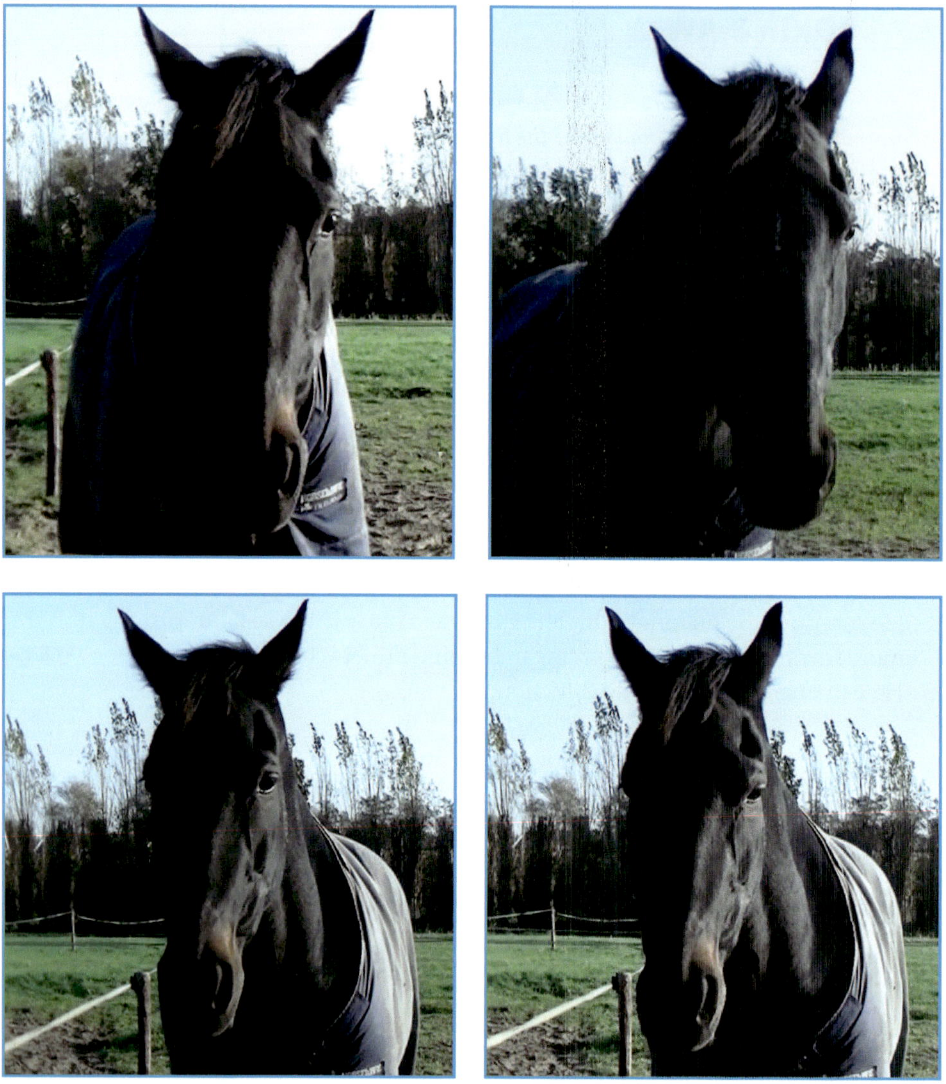

Figs 2.33–2.36 ***Top left:*** The horse looks at the person filming. ***Top right:*** The horse looks away as a calming signal. ***Bottom left:*** The horse looks away by turning his gaze inward, while also having turned his head a fraction. His eyes are half closed. ***Bottom right:*** The horse maintains his inward gaze and also half closes his eyes as a calming signal. These signals are meant for the person filming him at that moment.

An example of looking away by changing the direction of the gaze is also shown (**Figs 2.37, 2.38**).

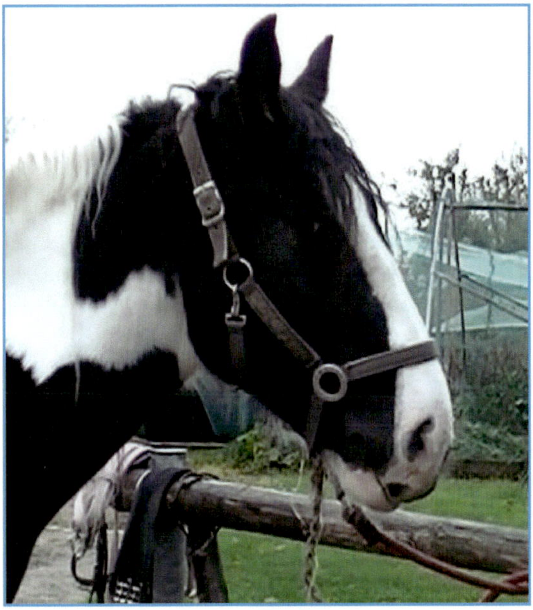

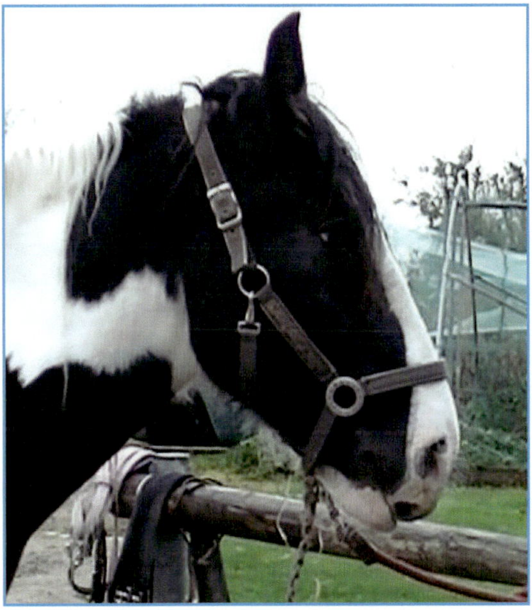

Figs 2.37, 2.38 *Top:* Here Koda is looking at the photographer. ***Bottom:*** Just a second later, he looks away as a calming signal.

2.8 CHEWING

The biological function of chewing is undisputed. Rotating the lower jaw and mixing saliva into food grinds food down into smaller pieces, allowing it to be swallowed. This is what happens when a horse has food in his mouth.

Chewing as a calming signal is characterised by the same rotating movement of the lower jaw, possibly also producing sound. However, the horse does not have food in his mouth. With this type of chewing, the tongue is not yet visible.

Chewing can occur as a single calming signal, but it also occurs in combination with nearly every other calming signal, for example, blinking, head turn, and neck turn (**Figs 2.39–2.41**). If a horse is chewing as a calming signal, and the tension rises, you will often see this reflected in his facial features, for instance the eyes and nostrils become round and tense (**Fig. 2.42**). You may also find that with rising tension the chewing is succeeded by tongue out chewing, yawning, or a jaw stretch. These calming signals are explained further in later sections.

You will often see a horse chewing when he has had a tense jaw for a few seconds or longer. It may be that the horse has been motionless as he listened to or watched a stimulus that was unknown to him. His eyes and ears will have been pointed towards the area of interest, his nose flaring to catch scents, the eyes perhaps opened a little wider. The moment the horse directs his attention away from the exciting stimulus, you see him loosening his jaw by chewing, thereby also giving a calming signal to another or himself.

Licking and chewing may be a direct consequence of a dry mouth, which is caused by a rise in adrenaline level.[1] The chewing and licking stimulates the secretion of saliva. An example of chewing and shaking off, although it is debatable whether these are calming signals, is when you see a horse chewing after he has rolled with tense jaws and then shaken it off.

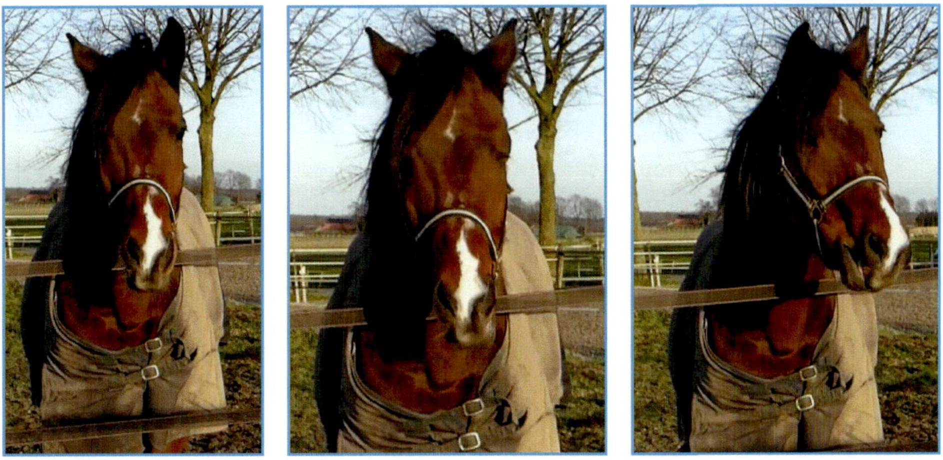

Figs 2.39–2.41 Merlin is being photographed face on. ***Left:*** Merlin looks at me and starts chewing as a calming signal for me, or to calm himself. I keep filming and facing him. ***Middle:*** His response is to still chew, but now he is also blinking his eyes. I change nothing about my posture. ***Right:*** Merlin gives a slightly stronger signal: he turns his head away slightly in an even more obvious calming signal. This is the head turn (there is no other stimulus he is watching or listening to). He keeps chewing. It is not until I turn away and increase the space between us that it stops.

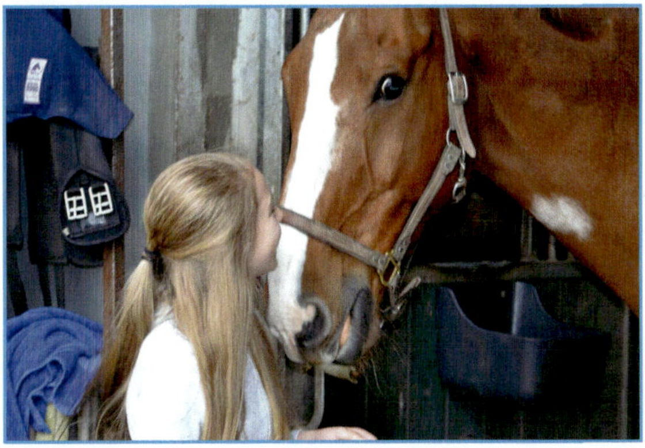

Fig. 2.42 Vosje is receiving attention from Anne, who is talking to him. A photographer is standing 2 metres away and takes a photo. At this moment, Vosje is chewing as a calming signal. It is unclear if he does this because Anne is standing close to him or because the photographer is causing him to feel tension. He looks directly at the photographer as he gives the calming signal, so it may be a combination of both. Other signs of tension are the very round nostrils and the round eye, the last being spread wide open in order to have a good view of the photographer.

NOTE: Horses do not produce saliva when they expect to get food. Dogs and people do.[2] If your horse gives calming signals when you are about to feed him, then the waiting is probably making him tense.

2.9 TONGUE OUT CHEWING

The movements made with tongue out chewing are the same as with the chewing described above. The horse makes a rotating motion with the lower jaw, possibly also producing sound. However, as he rotates his lower jaw, the tongue is pushed straight forward, out of the mouth, and then retracted again. This can happen several times in succession.

Tongue out chewing can be a first calming signal, but often it is seen when a number of other signals, such as blinking, lowering the head–neck position, and chewing, have already been given (**Figs 2.43, 2.44**). Tongue out chewing often functions as the next level after chewing. If the horse does not calm down, tongue out chewing may be followed by yawning or a jaw stretch, displacement behaviour, or stress signals.

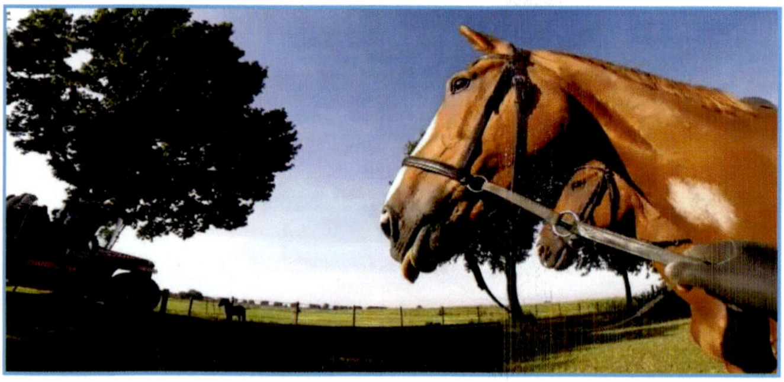

Fig. 2.43 A tractor passes by. The riders have dismounted. Vosje is standing in front. He is tongue out chewing. Orion is standing in the background. He is chewing, but his tongue is not showing. The direct stimulus causing the horses to show these calming signals is the tractor.

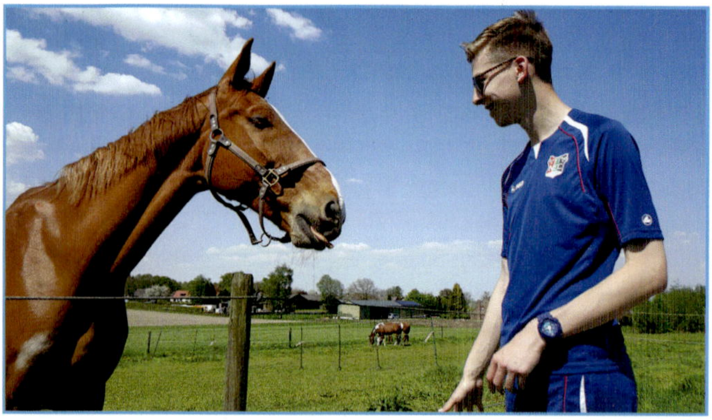

Fig. 2.44 Vosje is making calming signals at Sybrand. You can see him blinking and tongue out chewing.

CHEWING WITH THE TONGUE IN ORDER TO TASTE OR WHERE THERE IS PAIN

The nasal mucosa, the vomeronasal organ, and the taste buds on the tongue work closely together when a horse wishes to identify an incentive by smell and taste and get to know it better.[1] I have assumed that the horse in **Figs 2.45** and **2.46** is tongue out chewing for that purpose, tasting and smelling the odorant molecules emanating from the plastic clown. In this situation, chewing with the tongue sticking out follows directly after the sniffing and smelling of the object.

You also see chewing and tongue out chewing in horses who are suffering from dental pain or are, for example, drinking cold water. They can show this during and after drinking. You will also see chewing in horses who have just eaten something delicious and are still licking and chewing afterwards. In this situation it seems to be about prolonging the taste sensation and not about giving a calming signal. Also, the tongue will pass sideways along the lips.

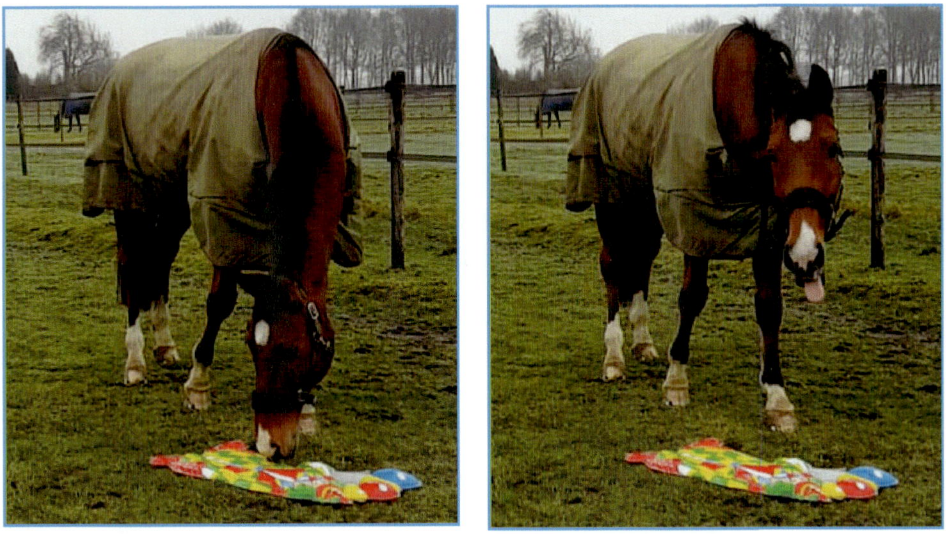

Figs 2.45, 2.46 Chewing with the tongue out.

2.10 YAWNING AND JAW STRETCH

YAWNING

When yawning, a horse opens his mouth for several seconds. The upper lip is retracted and the upper and lower teeth are visible. Sometimes the eyes roll back slightly or are half closed. The ears turn sideways during the yawn.

Yawning can be a signal of tiredness or a calming signal. Whenever I have observed yawning as a calming signal, it has happened when the horse is standing still; either he was already standing still or he stopped his walk to, among other things, yawn.

Can you tell the difference between a yawn that is a calming signal and a yawn that is a sign of tiredness? If the yawn is a calming signal, you will often see it show up as part of a pattern of other calming signals. Yawning as a sign of tiredness is a single signal (**Figs 2.47, 2.48**). It also occurs, for example, when the horse is lying down. I have not seen this when the yawn is a calming signal.

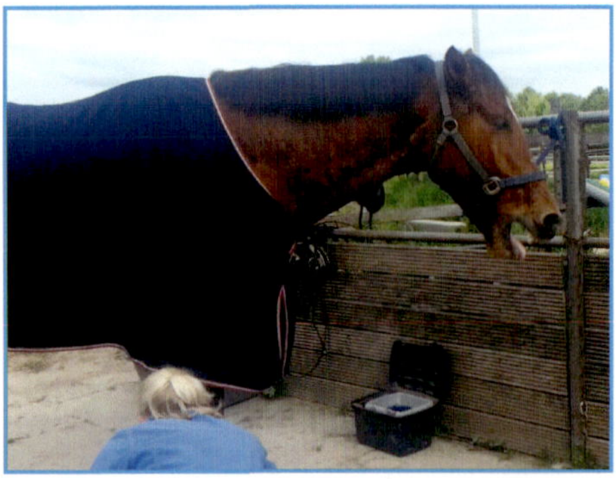

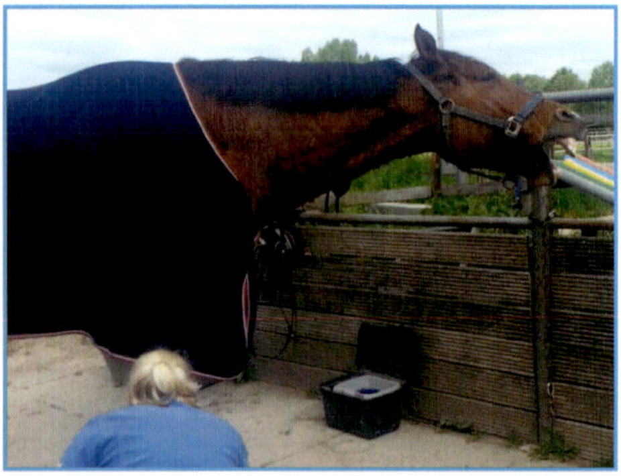

Figs 2.47, 2.48 Miranda is caring for Que Passa's hooves after riding. I am filming. Que Passa shows several calming signals, including a yawn. Why does he give calming signals? Maybe in response to me filming, or to having to stand still, or the treatment of his hoof. Had he yawned without other calming signals having preceded it, his yawn could have been a sign of tiredness.

JAW STRETCH

A jaw stretch is a calming signal that is sometimes used alone, but more often will be seen in combination with yawning. This can be both before and after the yawn. During a jaw stretch, the horse opens his mouth without uncovering his teeth. In addition, the tongue does not protrude. The mouth stays open for a few seconds, then closes again. The eyes are half closed or closed. The ears can be in any position, but I have most often seen the ears turned sideways or back.

You often see a jaw stretch as a follow-up to other calming signals such as blinking, looking away, chewing or tongue out chewing. Then, immediately afterwards or after a few seconds, the horse does a jaw stretch (**Figs 2.49, 2.50**).

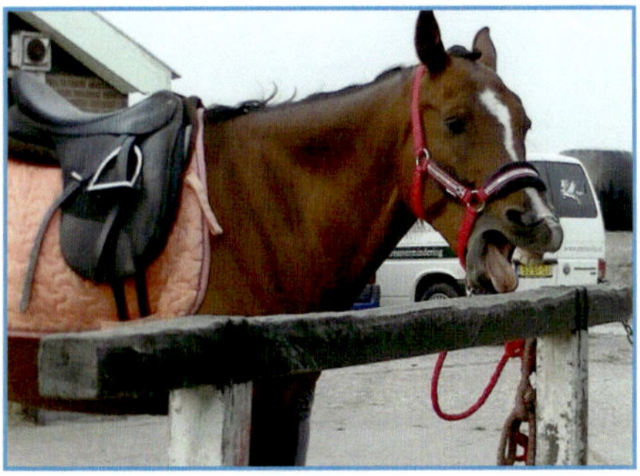
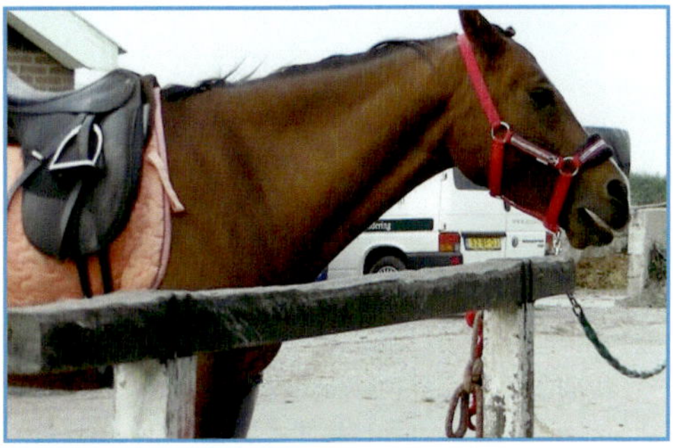

Figs 2.49, 2.50 Protect is showing a series of calming signals when he is being saddled. He chews, he tongue out chews, then he yawns (left), and finally he shows a jaw stretch (right). Note his half-closed eyes, also a calming signal.

Chewing, tongue out chewing, jaw stretch, and yawning also occur just before a rider puts on a bridle with bit (**Figs 2.51, 2.52**). Another example of a jaw stretch accompanied by other signals is shown in **Figs 2.53–2.56**. Sometimes, normal behaviour can be mistakenly interpreted as a jaw stretch (**Fig. 2.57**).

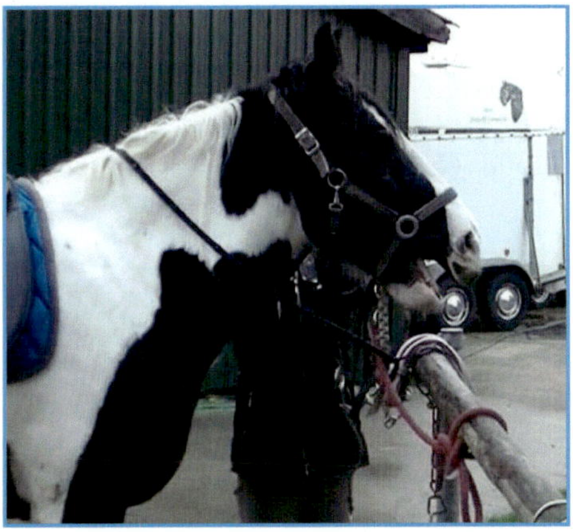
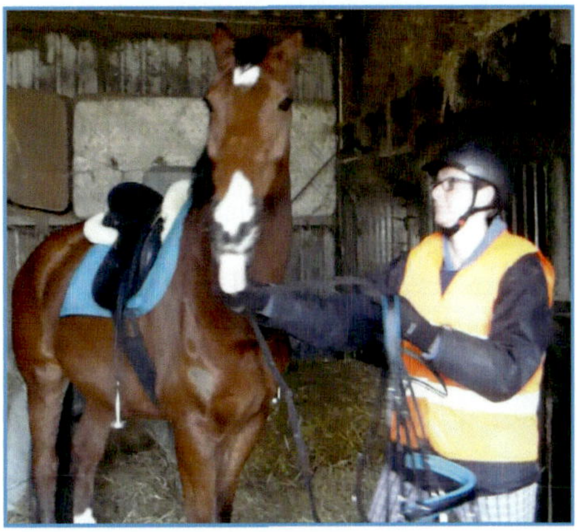

Figs 2.51, 2.52 Signals just before a bridle with bit is put on.

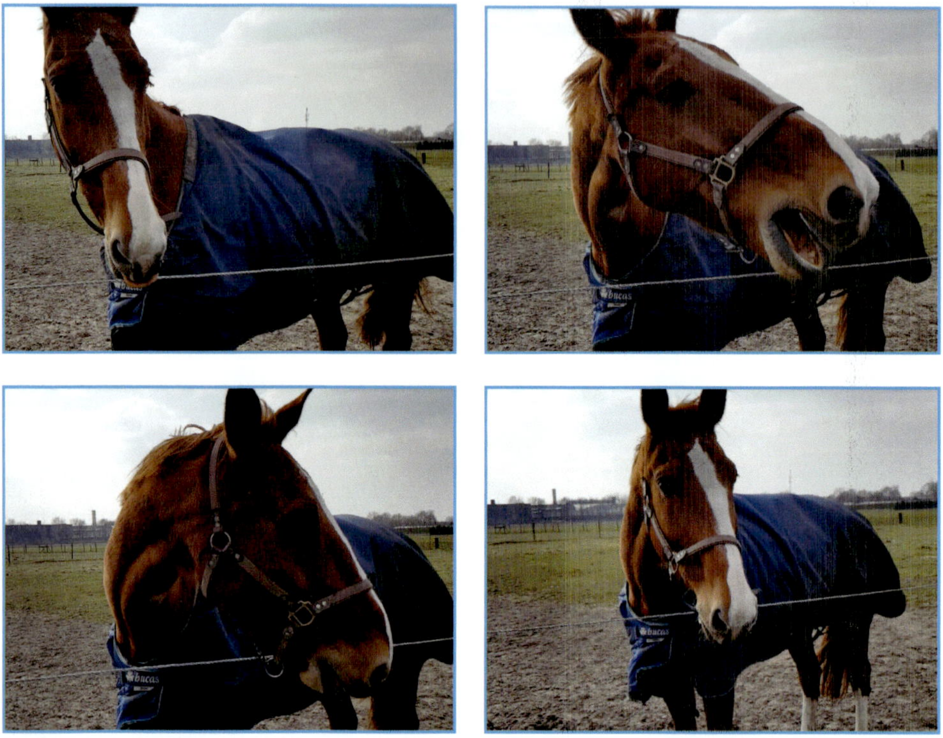

Figs 2.53–2.56 ***Top left:*** Vosje makes contact by looking at me. As a calming signal, he tongue out chews. ***Top right:*** Vosje shows a big jaw stretch. ***Bottom left:*** Vosje shows a neck turn, including turning away of the eyes (there is no stimulus in the direction he is looking). His right ear stays pointed at me. ***Bottom right:*** Vosje makes eye contact again.

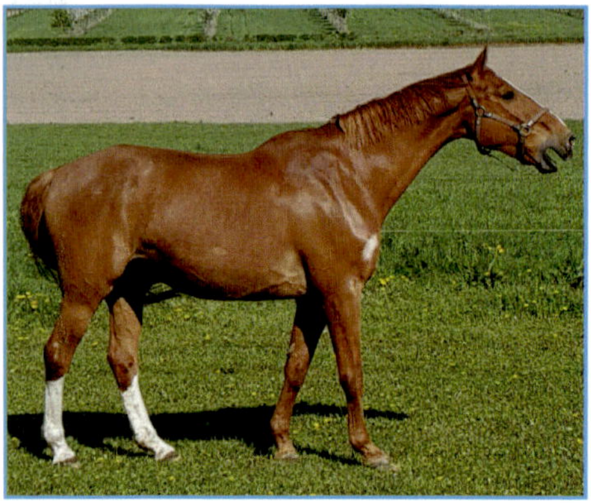

Fig. 2.57 In this photo Vosje is whinnying at the other horses. Without such a sound, it looks like a jaw stretch, but the difference is in the level of contact being made. Vosje's eyes are open and his ears are pointed forward. He is calling out to the other horses. His eyes show a very different picture to the half-closed eyes seen with a jaw stretch.

2.11 HEAD TURN

A horse makes a head turn when he turns his head to the side while his neck and body remain stationary. That is how you can recognise a head turn. A horse can make a head turn while walking, trotting, or standing still. I have seen it most often when horses are standing still. In a head turn the head turns to the left or right, according to the horse's preference, but always away from the stimulus he wants to appease or communicate with. Both ears face forward and turn along with the direction of the head. However, in some cases the horse points one ear forward and the other ear in the direction of the stimulus. During a head turn, eye contact with the stimulus is broken.

During a head turn, the horse may also display other calming signals that involve the head, such as blinking, chewing, tongue out chewing, yawning, or doing a jaw stretch. A head turn can occur in all body postures, although I have most often seen it in the mid-high and high positions.

With a head turn it is very clearly visible that the horse is communicating with the stimulus, for example, a person. After a head turn he swivels his head back to the forward position. He looks at the person, seemingly waiting for a response (**Figs 2.58–2.62**). Head turns can also occur when horses come into contact with each other for the first time (**Figs 2.63–2.66**).

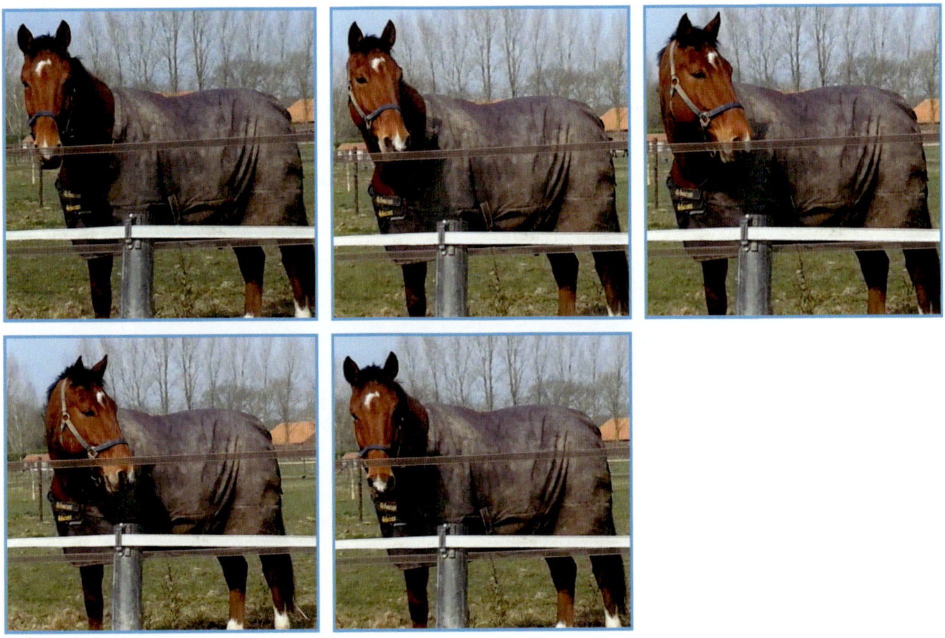

Figs 2.58–2.62 Que Passa is at pasture. I am on the other side of the barrier, fully facing him, holding the camera in front of me. In the top three photos, you can see him executing a head turn. On the film footage (not in the photos) you can also see him blinking several times during the head turn. In the last photo you see him coming back out of the head turn. He looks at me and my reaction to the head turn.

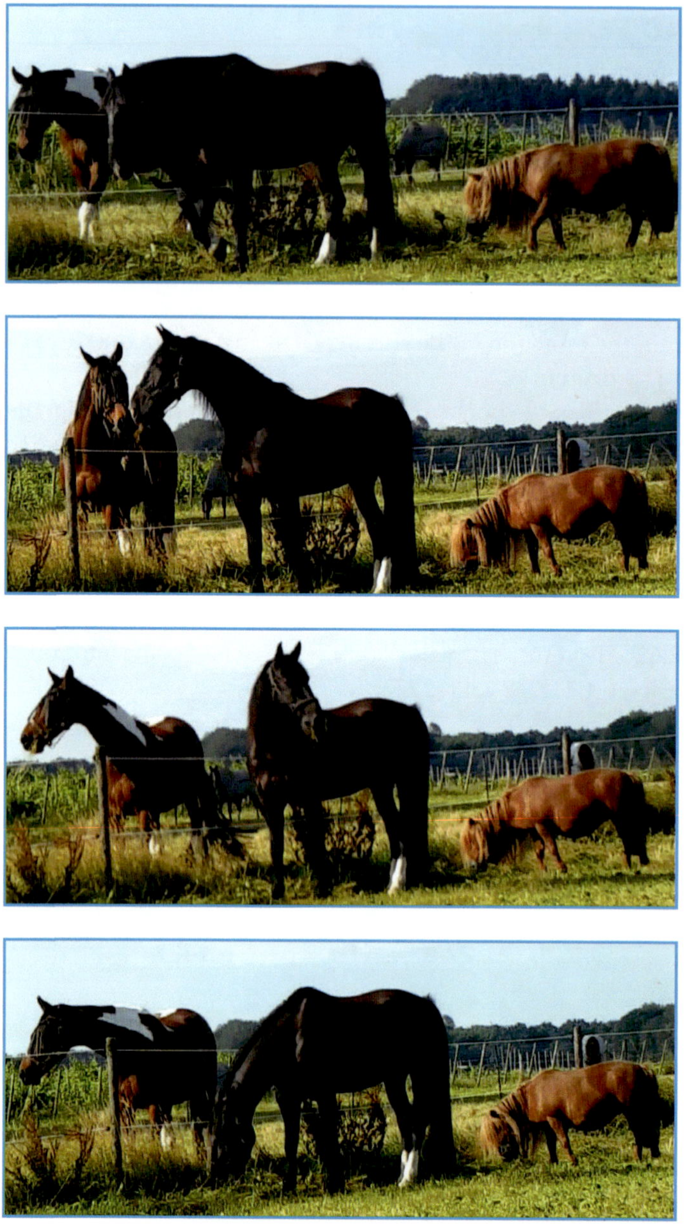

Figs 2.63–2.66 Victor (the dark bay horse on the right) and Saar (the horse on the far left) are paddock neighbours for the first time. Their greeting is very polite and appeasing. ***Top:*** They walk parallel to one another. ***Upper middle:*** They sniff at each other's noses. Victor has also half closed his eyes – a calming signal. Saar does a head turn as a calming signal. ***Lower middle:*** Victor does a head and neck turn. ***Bottom:*** Victor starts to eat. On the video film you can see Saar follow his example a second later. The eating as well as the showing of flanks are also calming signals, which will be explained further in sections 2.19 and 2.20.

When a person stands in front of a horse and faces it, the horse may perform a head turn as a calming signal (**Fig. 2.67**).

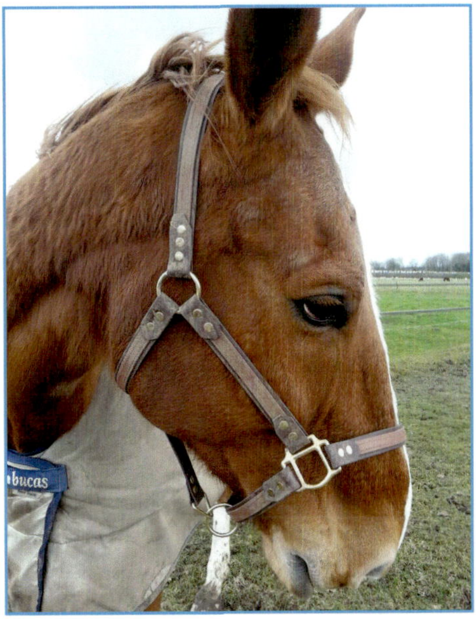

Fig. 2.67 A head turn as a calming signal. The ear is pointed at the person the horse is communicating with. Also, the eye is looking away, an additional calming signal. He is otherwise relaxed. The lower lip is loose and relaxed and protrudes slightly in front of the upper lip.

NOTE: During a head turn as a calming signal, there is nothing to be seen in the direction in which the horse is turning his head. This is fundamentally different to a horse who turns his head to look at something, in which you might also see a subtle weight change as can be seen in the photos in the Appendix (**Figs A1.3–A1.7**).

A HEAD TURN, BUT DIFFERENT

When you are spending time with your horse you may see a head turn that is motivated by something other than calming. Three motivations are listed below:

1 Head turn to follow or look at another stimulus (**Fig. 2.68**).
2 Head turn to show where the horse wants to go.
3 The horse turns his head towards you and back to invite you to join him when walking away (fig. 2.72).

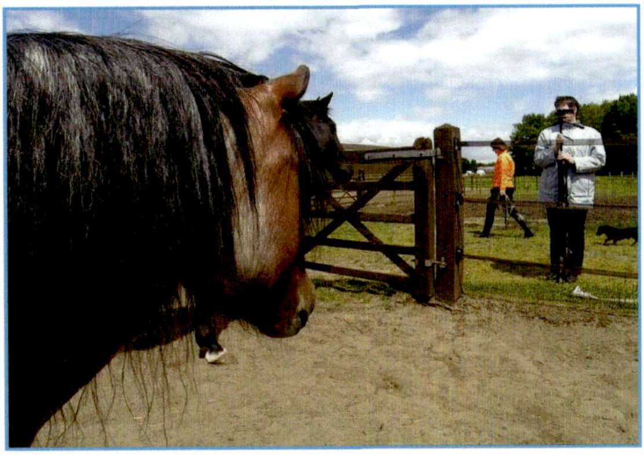

Fig. 2.68 I am standing at Indy's right shoulder, petting him. Indy turns his head away from me and uses his eyes and ears to follow a person who passes by outside the arena. This head turn is not a calming signal to me, but an examination of a new stimulus. You can see that both his eyes and ears are pointed at this new stimulus.

Of course, it is possible for both 2 and 3 to occur at the same time; the horse may use a head turn as a calming signal and also to indicate where he wants to go. In this situation he very clearly looks in a particular direction (**Figs 2.69–2.71**).

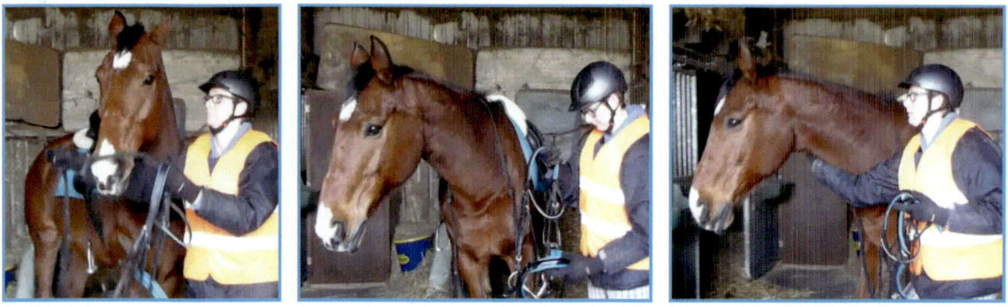

Figs 2.69–2.71 Orion turns away from his owner, using a head turn. His ears are pointed back and initially reflect a flight movement. A second later, this is indeed what happens. He moves away a few paces, one ear still turned back and the other pointed at where he is going.

WHAT ARE YOU DOING? ARE YOU COMING ALONG (FIG. 2.72)?

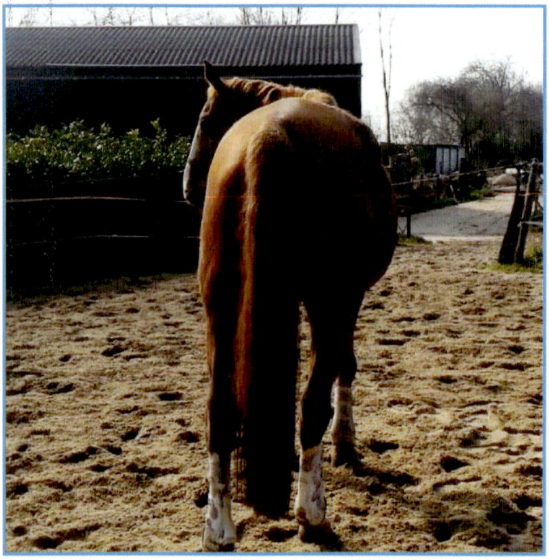

Fig. 2.72 Vosje is walking towards the gate of the arena. His right ear is pointed to where he is going. His body walks straight forward. He turns his head and looks at me out of his left eye. His left ear is also pointed at me. I have seen this posture a lot in horses who are walking away from the group. After looking back, his head is somewhere between the horizontal and mid-high positions. The other horses follow. It seems to be an invitation or a check to see if others are following.

2.12 NECK TURN

A neck turn as a calming signal is more clearly visible than a head turn, looking away, blinking, or half closing the eyes. In a neck turn, not only is the head turned away from the stimulus with which the horse is communicating, but the whole neck bends as well. The torso and feet remain in the same fixed position. The horse is not turning his neck to look at another object (see **Fig. 2.119**). Both ears are turned forward, or one ear faces forward and the other is pointed at who or what has grabbed the horse's attention.

A neck turn often occurs in combination with a head turn, in which case it follows a head turn as a calming signal. First the horse shows a head turn. Then he rotates back to whoever or whatever he is communicating with. After that he shows a neck turn (**Figs 2.73, 2.74**). During a neck turn, a horse may also show other head-related calming signals, such as perhaps blinking, chewing, tongue out chewing, yawning, or doing a jaw stretch. I have seen a neck turn when horses are walking and when they are standing still.

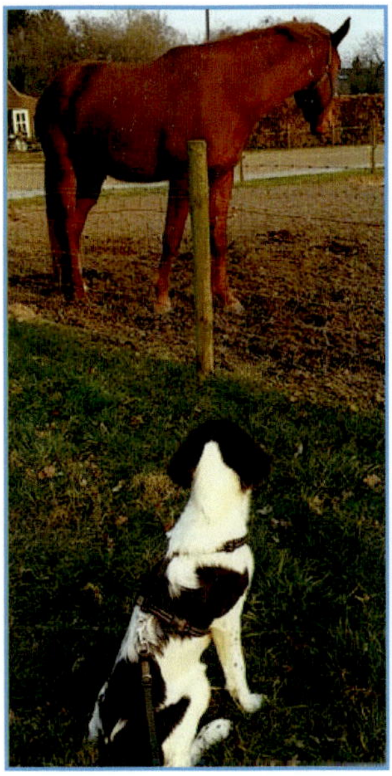

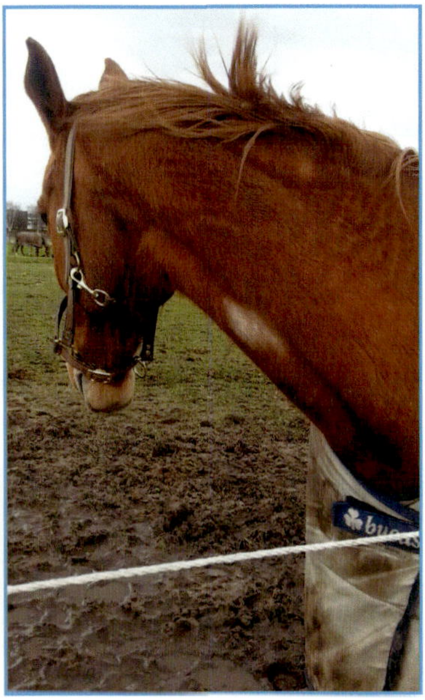

Figs 2.73, 2.74 Both these horses show multiple calming signals in relation to a new stimulus. ***Left:*** The horse is making a neck turn as a calming signal to the dog. ***Right:*** The horse makes a neck turn to the photographer. Also note the position of the ears. Both horses have one ear aimed at the source of their interest – the dog and the photographer.

*Gertie and Hanneke are out for a ride. They meet at a crossroads. The horses have seen one another once before, 6 months earlier. Orion, the horse on the left (**Fig. 2.75**), walks into view. The horses then look at each other (**Fig. 2.76**). Then, in turn, they each do a head and neck turn, calming one another and themselves (**Figs 2.77, 2.78**). A polite start to the proceedings. The reins on both horses hang loose. Gertie and Hanneke talk to each other and do not interfere with their horses (**Fig. 2.79**).*

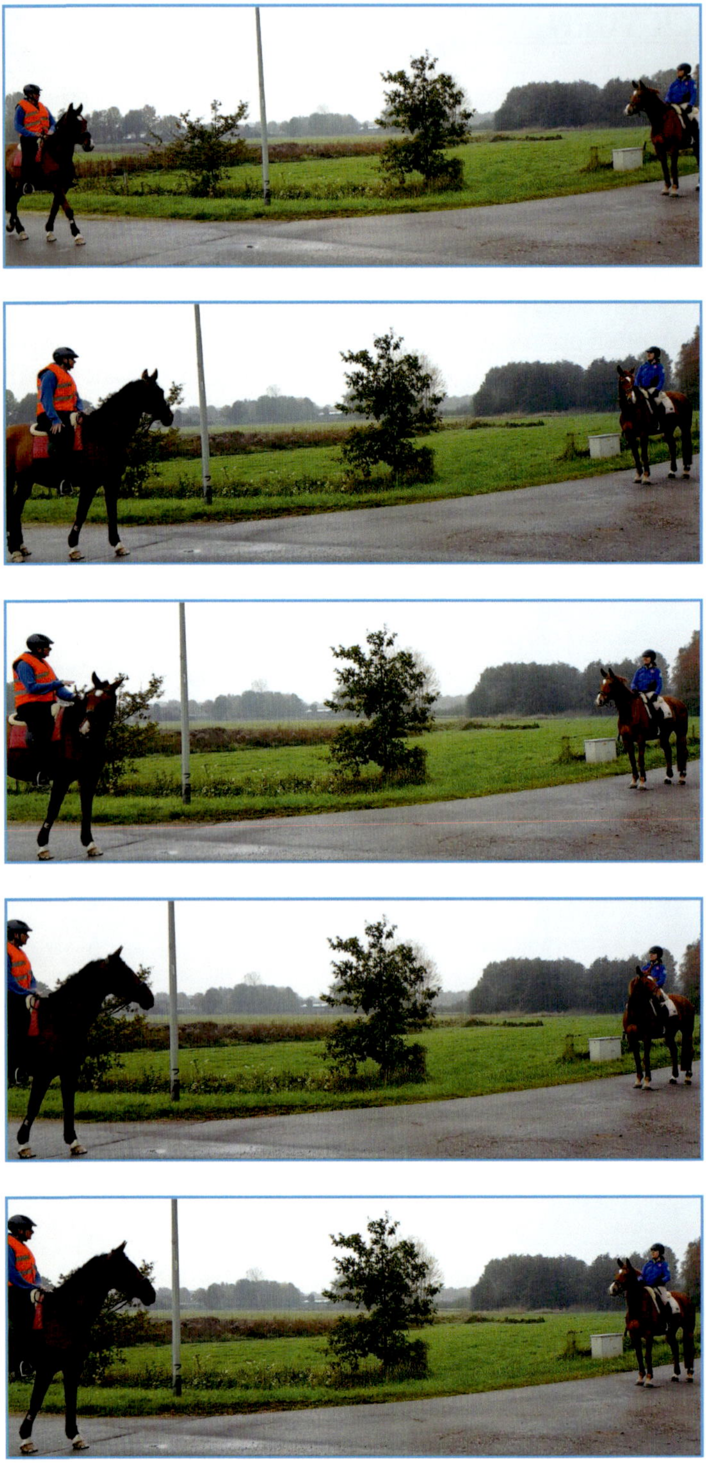

Figs 2.75–2.79 A meeting of two horses.

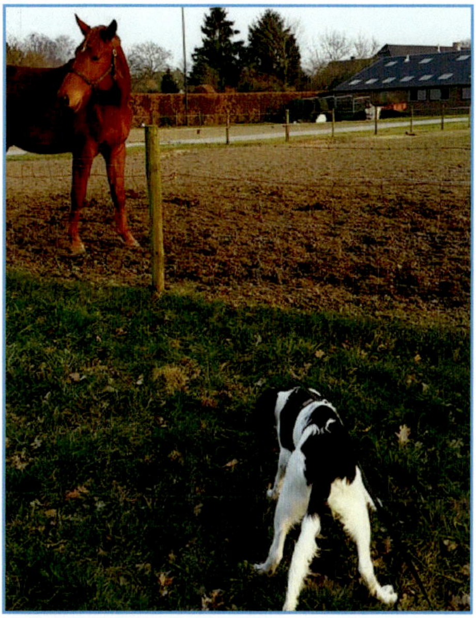

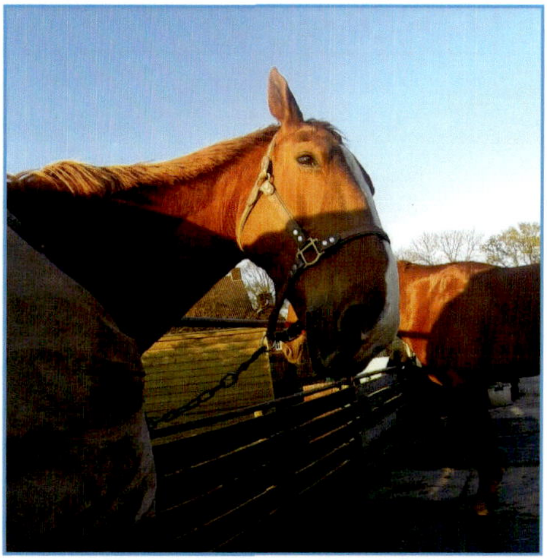

Figs 2.80, 2.81 Both horses turn their head and neck to have a look at something.

NOTE: A horse may also turn his neck and head in order to have a good look at something. In this situation it is a self-contained motion with the aim of looking. The focus of his eyes is then actually turned outwards to see, not necessarily to communicate (**Figs 2.80, 2.81**). But of course, both at the same time is also possible (i.e. communicating with someone while simultaneously checking out who he is communicating with). If that is the case, you will see the horse take a good look at a person, animal, or object from within a sequence of calming signals.

2.13 NECK SHAKE

During a neck shake, the horse's torso stays still. His head and neck are between the horizontal and mid-high positions. The horse pushes his nose forwards. His neck and head move in a short, side-to-side shaking motion a number of times. During a sideways shake, the eyes are closed. A neck shake can occur as part of a sequence of calming signals, in which case it is often used as a next-level signal. However, it can also be regarded as a single calming signal, used as a direct response to an action that has caused tension in the horse (**Figs 2.82–2.85**). A neck shake is one of the calming signals that I believe indicates that the horse feels tension or has felt tension.

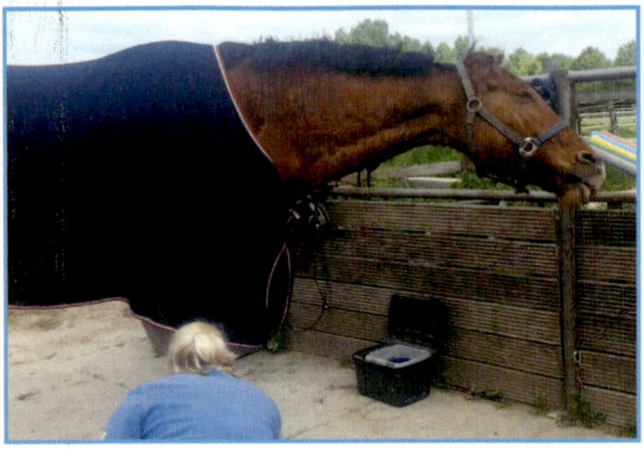

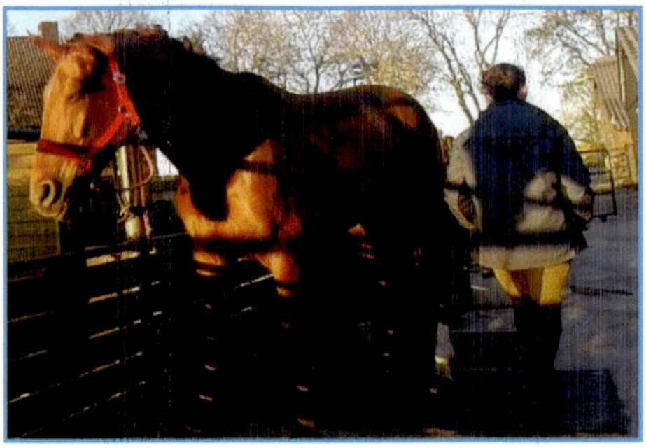

Figs 2.82, 2.83 ***Left:*** I am filming Que Passa as he is being cared for by his owner. Que Passa shows multiple calming signals: a yawn, a jaw stretch, and this neck shake. ***Right:*** Hanneke has just dried the foreleg. In response to this, Elanta shows a neck shake as a calming signal, something she is prone to doing after Hanneke has cared for her feet.

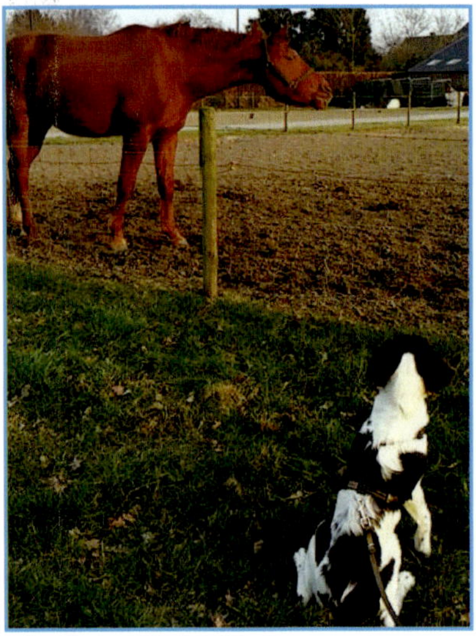

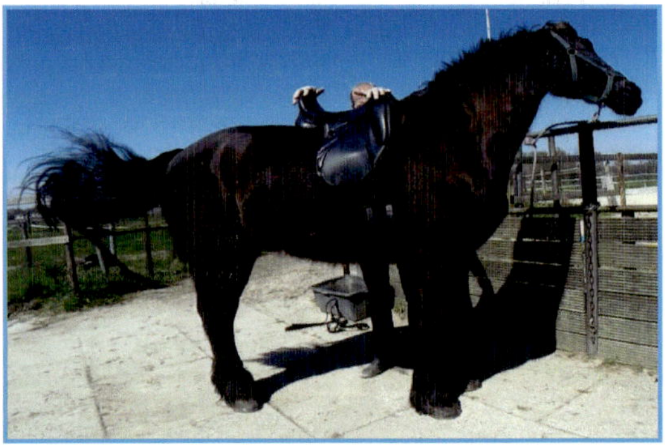

Figs 2.84, 2.85 ***Left:*** This horse shows a number of calming signals in relation to the dog, one of which is a neck shake. ***Right:*** Itske shows a neck shake when the saddle is put on his back for fitting purposes. He also flicks his tail.

A neck shake can also have a biological function, for example, when a horse wants to shake off flies, sand, or water.

2.14 BODY SHAKE

A body shake is executed from a stationary position. The horse lowers his head and neck to a horizontal or mid-low position. The nose is extended forwards slightly. He makes a sideways shaking motion with his body, starting at his head, then moving to his neck, his torso, and finally flowing into his tail (**Figs 2.86, 2.87**). Sometimes the mouth is slightly open during this shaking.

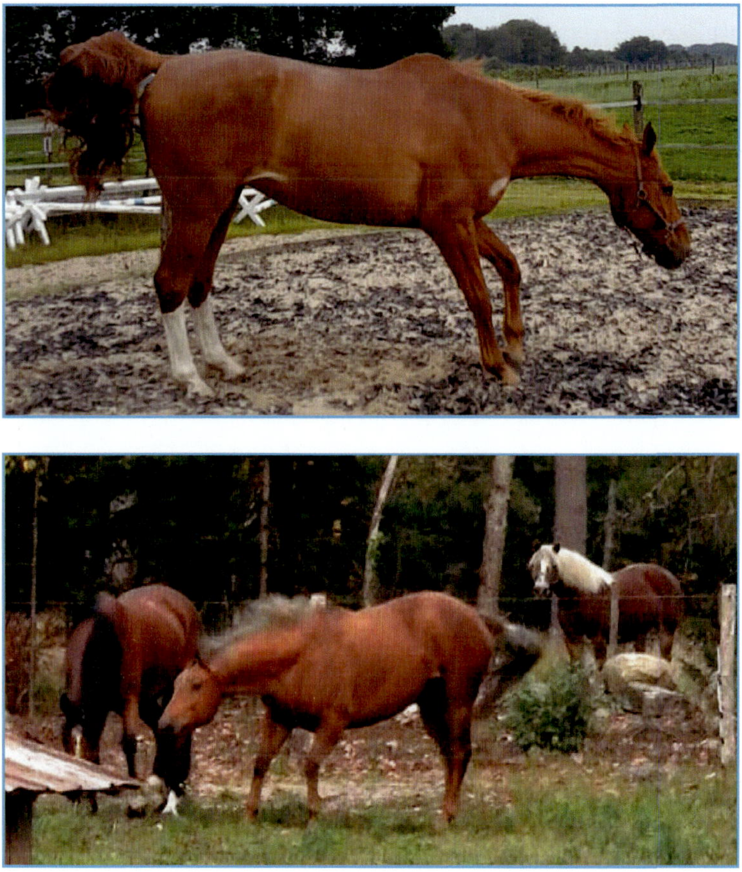

Figs 2.86, 2.87 A body shake.

As a calming signal, a body shake can occur in two ways:

1 As a single signal, in which case it is a direct response to a stimulus that has caused tension in the horse or is part of a sequence.
2 If the body shake is part of a sequence of calming signals, you will often have already seen a number of other calming signals before it is the body shake's turn. The body shake often follows a neck shake.

I see Prince walking towards the end of the paddock. He wants to eat grass by ducking his head underneath an electrified fence. He touches the fence and receives a shock. He backs up forcefully and expels a powerful puff of air. Then he does a body shake. He walks away from the fence and does a neck shake. His neck is in a horizontal position, his eyes are half closed, and his ears are pointed forwards. He turns towards the fence. He shows a see-saw lowering in relation to the fence, ears pointed back. Then he does another see-saw lowering (see section 2.15) towards the fence, eyes half closed, ears forward, and he repeats the see-saw lowering again, eyes half closed, ears forward, finally doing a neck shake. Then Prince holds his head in the horizontal position, eyes half closed, ears pointed sideways, and nostrils long and relaxed.

This scenario lasted for a minute and 5 seconds. In that time we have one body shake, two neck shakes, and three instances of half-closed eyes. The see-saw lowering is debatable. It is possible that Prince is simply having another good look at the fence and, in doing so, changes his perspective by lowering and raising his head.[3] It can also be a calming signal or, of course, both. But those are a lot of signals in just 1 minute!

Elanta is tied up outside. Her owner is grooming her. She walks away to fetch something. Elanta stands alone as I observe her. Then a farmer emerges from around the corner, pushing a small mower. Elanta looks over and immediately does a body shake.

People are also familiar with this phenomenon. Have you ever taken a bite of something that is generally considered delicious, but that you then find utterly disgusting? In this situation, the chances are you have to suppress a full body shiver too.

Just like a neck shake, a body shake also has a biological function. Shaking allows the horse, for example, to get rid of sand, water, or annoying flies. So it makes sense that you often see horses do a body shake after they have been rolling. Whether a body shake can also be a calming signal in that situation is an interesting question.

2.15 LOWERING OF THE HEAD AND NECK

When the horse lowers his head and neck as a calming signal, you will see him move his head and neck from a high, mid-high, or horizontal position to a mid-low or low position, and then back up to a mid-high to high position. The amount of time during which the lowered posture is maintained varies. If the head moves down and right back up again, I call this a see-saw lowering. If, however, the lowered pose is held for 5 seconds or longer, I call it a sustained lowering.

SEE-SAW LOWERING

In 1 second, the head goes from a high, mid-high, or horizontal position to a mid-low to a low position. Then, within 1 to 5 seconds, the head is lifted back up to a mid-high or high position. The horse can do this while standing still, walking, trotting, or cantering.

You may see see-saw lowering as a single calming signal in direct response to a stimulus. For example, if a horse has trouble lifting one particular leg, he may show a see-saw lowering just before it is that leg's turn to be lifted. See-saw lowering also occurs as part of a sequence of calming signals.

I also often see see-saw lowering when horses see a new object, animal, or person. The lowering and then raising can have a dual purpose here. It can have a calming effect on the stimulus in question and on the horse itself. It can also enable the horse to view the stimulus from a different perspective. In her book *Horse Senses,* Susan McBane explains:

'The field of vision of horses consists of a horizontal band of their best acuity in comparison with the circular spot of best acuity found in humans. This is due to a 'visual streak' just below the equator of the retina. [...] The horse's eye does not move far or easily in its bony socket (unlike the eye of humans) and this characteristic, plus the poor accommodation and the visual streak, means the horse has to move his head around, up and down and from side to side a good deal to bring objects onto the visual streak and obtain the best view possible. It is not the case of the horse having to focus objects onto a ramp-shaped retina, as was previously thought, but of him needing to manoeuvre his head and therefore his eyes and visual streaks into the best position to capture the image he is trying to look at'.[3]

A see-saw lowering often occurs after a horse has seen, heard, or experienced something exciting and perhaps a little scary. It almost seems as if by quickly lowering his head, he is letting the tension slide off himself. You will sometimes hear a horse snorting briefly during a see-saw lowering.

Letting tension slide off is also relevant when a horse has been experiencing higher tension for a little while or has been spooked. When the tension level start to drop, that is when you will see the horse do a see-saw lowering. If the tension is high, he will even do it during a trot or canter. The downward position can be held for a few seconds in that case. If the tension gradually starts to drop, you will see other calming signals (**Figs 2.88–2.91**). If, however, the tension lingers a bit, the see-saw lowering may be interspersed with signs of tension or displacement activities, or both.

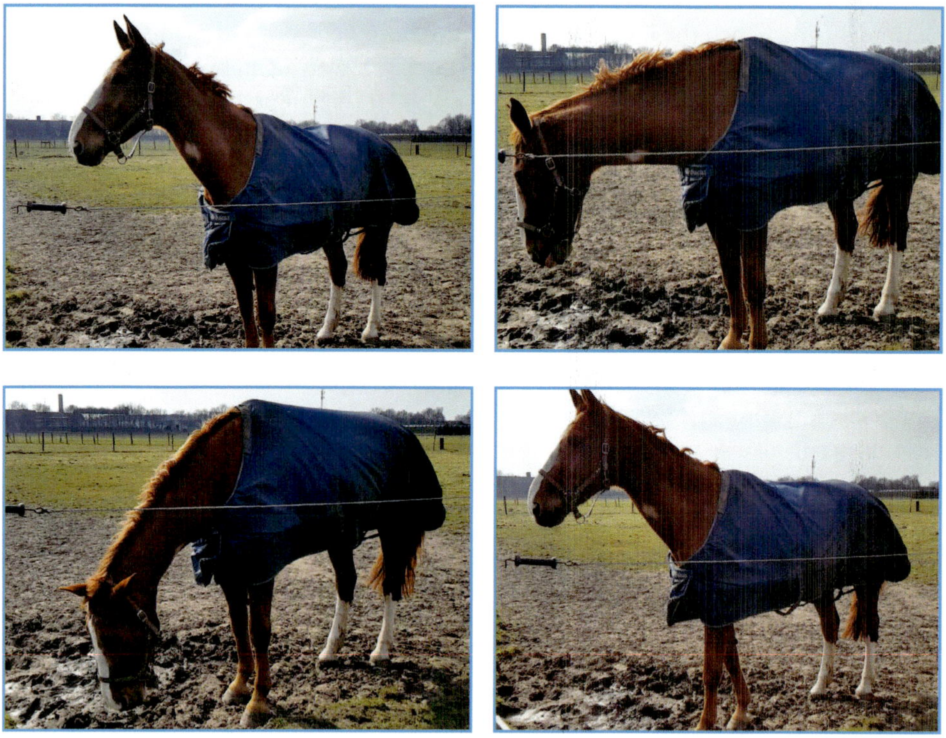

Figs 2.88–2.91 ***Top left:*** Vosje has to wait and looks in the direction he wants to go. ***Top right:*** He lowers his head and neck as a calming signal while also tongue out chewing and blinking. ***Bottom left:*** Vosje lowers his head and raises it again immediately afterwards. ***Bottom right:*** Vosje looks in the direction he wants to go (see section 5.10).

SUSTAINED LOWERING

In sustained lowering as a calming signal, the horse moves his head and neck from a high, mid-high, or horizontal position to a mid-low to low position in a single second. This pose is held for a minimum of 5 seconds, but can even be held for 25 seconds or more, after which the head is lifted to a mid-high to high position again. I have seen sustained lowering in horses who are communicating with familiar horses (**Fig. 2.92**), other animals, or people. You also see it when, for instance, a horse is being led into a paddock that already has a number of horses in it. As he is being walked into the paddock, the horse maintains a lowered head and neck position. This sustained lowering is a calming signal for the others

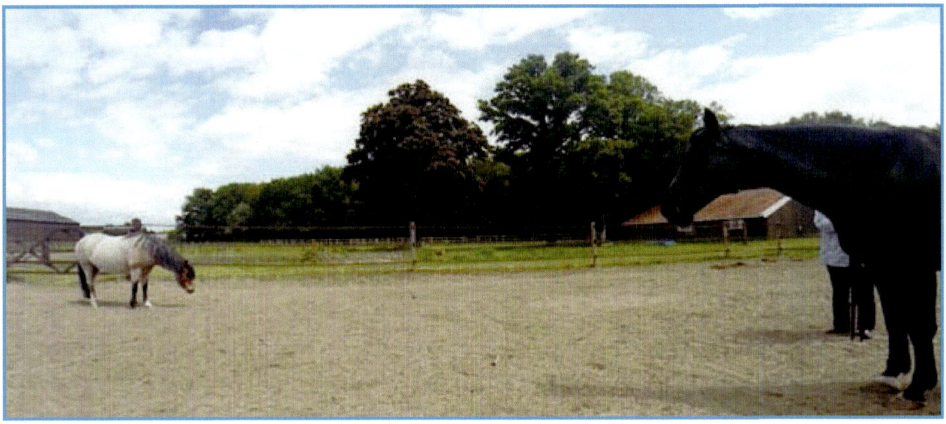

Fig. 2.92 Sustained lowering.

and possibly also for himself. The sustained lowering can also be expanded with a head or neck turn. I have mostly seen sustained lowering during a walk or a stand still.

I have also seen this sustained lowering in horses who were going into a shut-down mode (see section 4.4) and who were closing themselves off from stimuli in the outside world.

You also see a lowering of the head and neck that is sustained for a long time in horses who are exposed to the elements, such as wind and rain, when at pasture. They can then turn their hindquarters into the wind and hold their heads lower.

Holding the head lower can also be seen in horses who are asleep or nodding off, and, of course, it is also seen in horses who are sniffing the ground for a good place to roll or to look for something. In these situations, the lowering of the head and neck is not a calming signal, but a necessary feature of other behaviour.

2.16 CURVING

Today I brought a blue, plastic, inflatable dolphin to the stables where my horse is boarded. Then, one at a time, I placed the dolphin in the paddocks of a number of horses, at a good distance from the horses themselves. The reactions were very different. Some horses were curious and wanted to see, smell, and feel the new object. Others adopted a wait and see strategy. They grazed for 10 minutes with their flanks facing the dolphin. This allowed them to see the object, but that was as far as they were willing to go.

When a horse wants to move towards a person, animal, or object carefully and politely, you will often see him making an arc. He will walk in a curved line from his original position to the stimulus he wants to approach. But it is not only his path that is curved; as he makes his arc, the horse can also curve his body slightly around its central axis. The size of the curve depends on the amount of room the horse has in relation to the stimulus, but also on the horse's assessment and how polite he wants to be as he approaches. As he walks his curved line, the horse may show other signals such as a head turn, blinking, a see-saw lowering, pausing, immobility, and slowing down (**Figs 2.93–2.98**) (see section 2.21).

Walking in a curve may also be combination of a calming signal and a way of looking at an object from a different angle, because it alternates the horse's view from binocular (using both eyes at once) to monocular (using only one eye).

WHEN DO YOU SEE HORSES APPROACH A PERSON, ANIMAL, OR OBJECT IN A STRAIGHT LINE?

- When they are confident about the person or object they are approaching.
- When they are confident in the good and close relationship they have with the person, animal, or object they are approaching.
- When they are playing.
- When they are fearful and looking for support.
- When they have been taught to do this through, for example, food rewards.
- When they are giving a distance increasing signal such as, for example, chasing away or air biting.
- When they are making a direct, frontal attack.

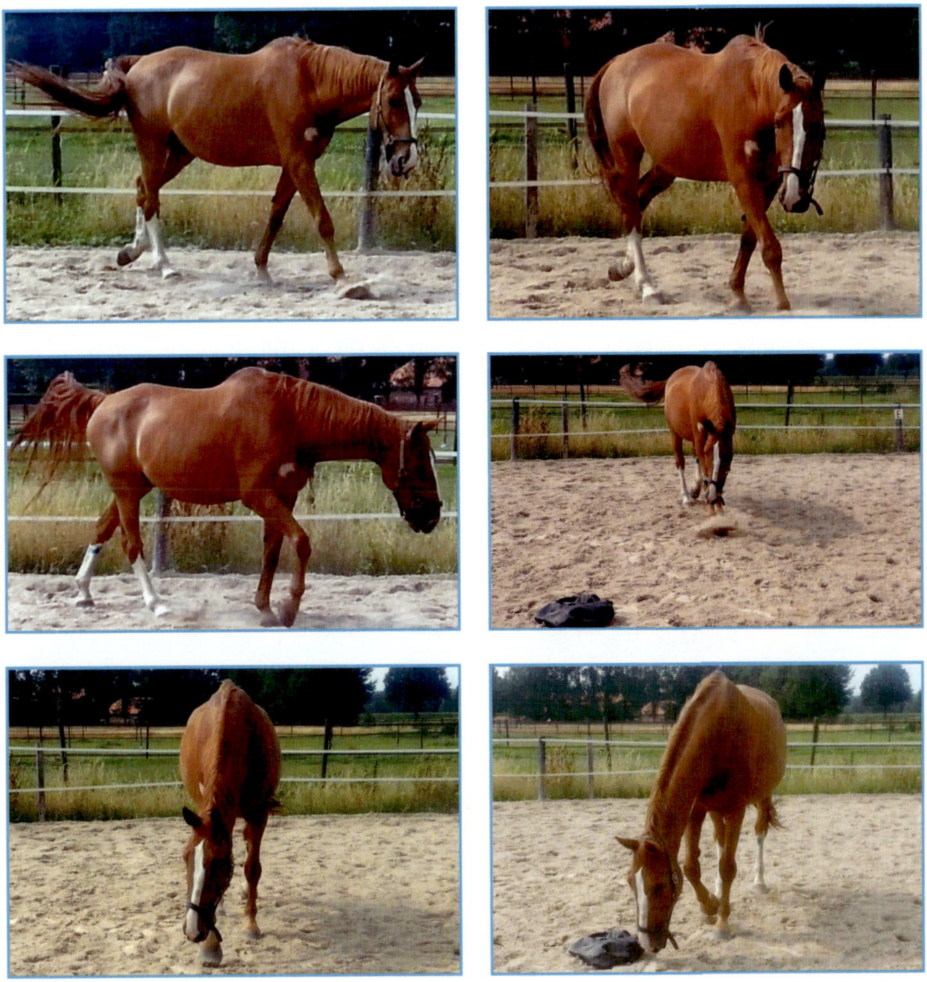

Figs 2.93–2.98 The arc is started from a horizontal head/neck position. The nostrils are not round but long and relaxed. During the arc, Vosje does a head turn and chews. This may be an added gesture of politeness towards the object or it may be Vosje trying to calm himself and releasing tension (or a combination of both). The head is turned back and the arc resumed until the object is reached. There were a lot of flies on the day I filmed this, so the tail movement is probably chasing off flies.

2.17 SPLITTING

Horses split when they want to prevent a possible conflict between two parties. When a horse splits, he changes position in order literally to form a barrier between two parties. These can be two other horses, a horse and a dog or other animal (**Figs 2.99–2.104**), a horse and a child, a horse and a cyclist, a horse and an object, or even a horse and a sound that is causing tension.

Splitting enables the horse to stop the two parties he is splitting up from continuing the behaviour they had initiated or intended (**Figs 2.105, 2.106**).

Horses can split by walking to the right strategic place and stopping there. However, you will also see splitting happening while a horse is walking, trotting, or cantering. He will then pass between two people, animals, or animals and objects in a walk, trot, or canter.

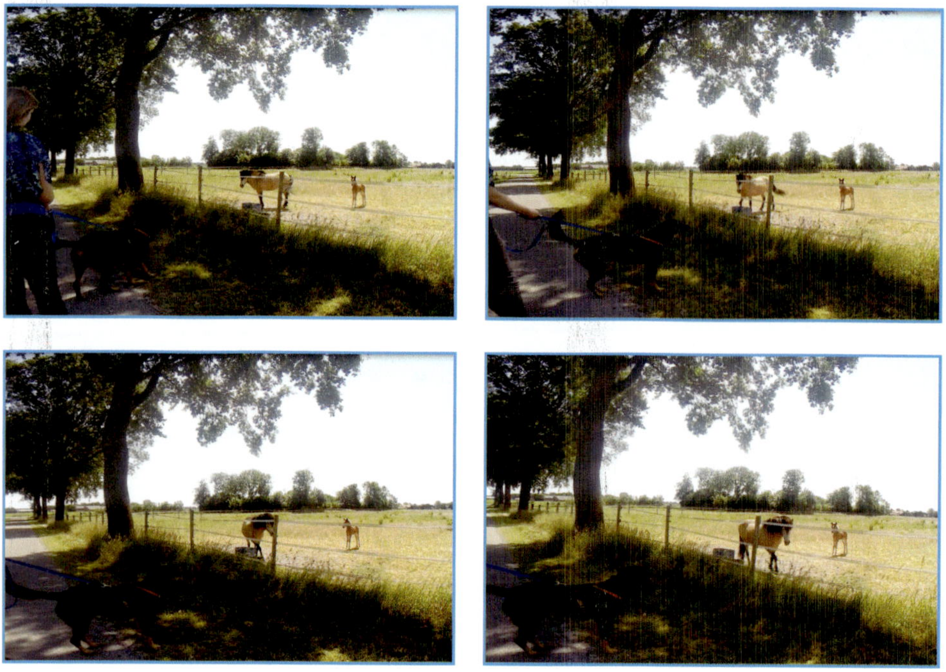

Figs 2.99–2.104 The dog and the foal are looking at one another across the paddock fence. The pony on the left wants to prevent possible conflict and splits up the dog and the foal. The foal's mother is watching from a distance. She remains off camera in these photos.

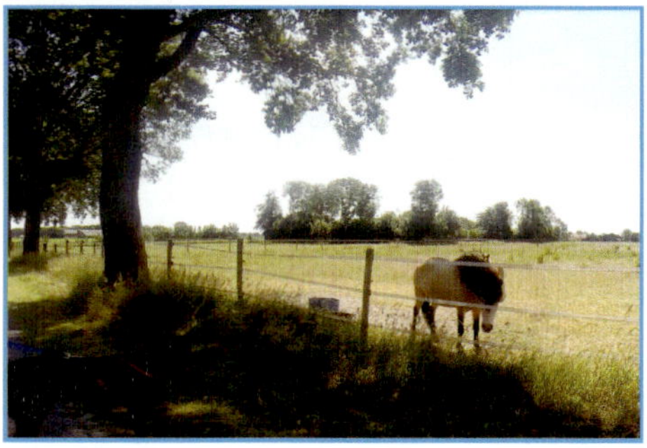

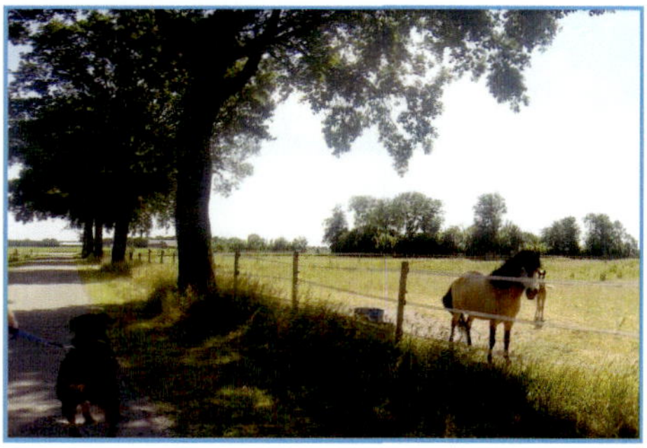

Figs 2.99–2.104 *(Continued)*

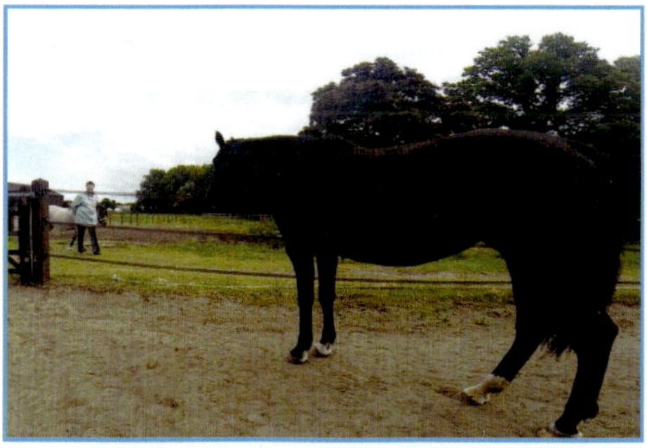

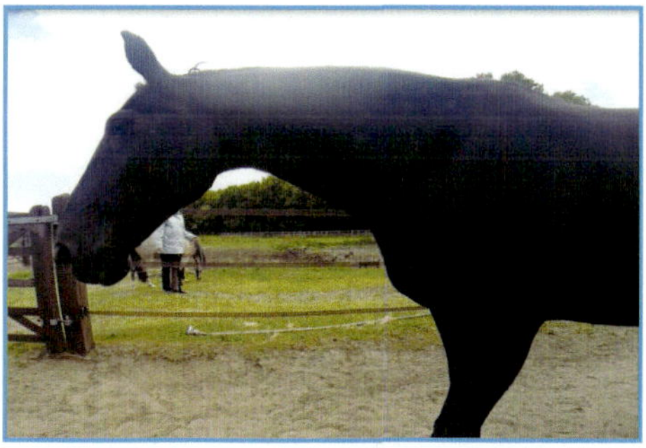

Figs 2.105, 2.106 In these photos I am filming and taking photos. While doing so I am talking to Ristin and fully facing her. Because of the distance, we are speaking a little loudly. In the left-hand photo, Pearl turns her left ear towards me. In the right-hand photo, she looks at me as well. Then she splits between Ristin and me. She moves between us, stops, and stays there for a few seconds before moving on.

SPLITTING IN ORDER TO GUARD OR PROTECT A VALUABLE POSSESSION

When a person, animal, or object has great value to a horse, he may try to keep it exclusive by splitting. The horse will then move in between the valuable item in question and another horse. You will often see this happening at pasture where, for example, there is not always enough water in the trough or when there is food in one place and it is not enough for all the horses. In these situations, the food and water are valuable items to commandeer.

Every horse attaches his own subjective value to people, animals, or objects. This value can differ depending on the individual horse; for example, you can drag one person out of bed in the middle of the night for a piece of whipped cream cake, but another person will not get up for anything except a morning walk.

If several horses attribute the same value to the same object, animal, or person, it can cause unrest. Depending on the strength of each horse's internal motivation and the item's worth, both horses may want to appropriate the object. How the horses handle this situation depends on the strength of their individual motivation, their determination, and their temperament, as well as on how long a conflict over a valuable animal, person, or object lasts. As such, splitting is also used in very tense situations in which you might also see distance increasing signals (see Chapter 3).

Horses who are split and accept this often respond with calming signals, such as chewing, doing a head or neck turn, or showing a see-saw lowering, or they turn their flank or backside towards the splitting horse and start to graze. This may be accompanied by a horizontal or mid-low head–neck position.

SPLITTING, BUT WITH LESS EMPHASIS

When a splitter does not have to emphasise his action, two forms of splitting may occur. The first is where you find the splitting horse in front of an imaginary line between the two parties he wants to split (**Fig. 2.107**). The second is when the splitting horse turns his hindquarters towards the imaginary line between the two parties he wants to split (**Fig. 2.108**). Although less obvious, the goal of the splitter stays the same. He wants to split the two parties to prevent escalations or he wants to split the parties to keep one of them for himself, because it has a high value for him. He can therefore step in quite quickly when he needs to emphasise his role as splitter.

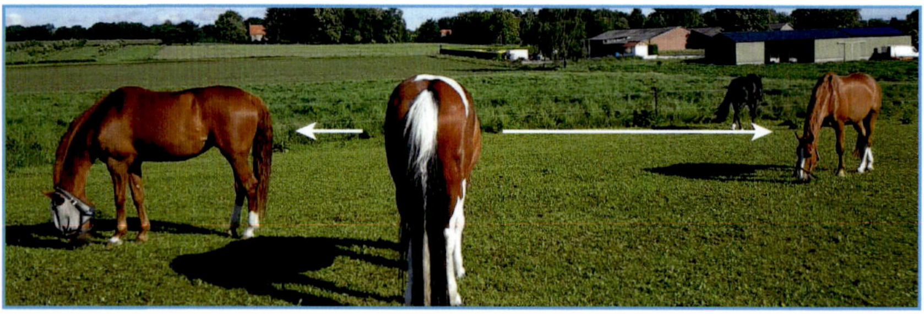

Fig. 2.107 Vosje is on the right. He is focused on Lorain, the chestnut mare on the left. His frontal positioning says he wants to go in her direction. Saar, the Paint Horse, is splitting the two by standing in front of the imaginary line between Vosje and Lorain.

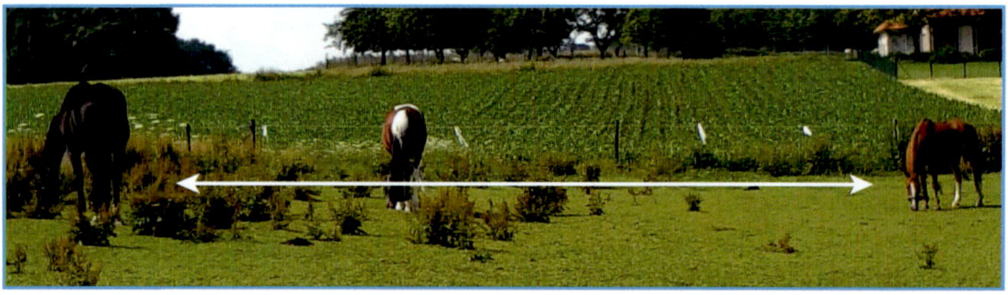

Fig. 2.108 Vosje is on the right in this photo. In the past weeks he has showed distance increasing signals (see section 3.8) towards Oscar, the black horse on the left. He has chased Oscar away on several occasions. Saar, the Paint Horse, has been Oscar's protector. She has been splitting Vosje and Oscar on a regular basis. After several weeks of this, she now starts to split in a less intense and obvious way between Vosje and Oscar. She turns her hindquarters towards the imaginary line between Vosje and Oscar. She can still see them both perfectly and can step in at any time if needed.

2.18 SHOWING THE HINDQUARTERS

To me it was a great eye opener to discover that how a horse stands and positions himself has a communicative meaning. I had never considered this before. There are two postures that, as calming signals, keep coming back under similar circumstances:

1 Standing so that the hindquarters face the other person or animal or the stressor.
2 Standing so that a flank faces the other person or animal or the stressor.

First I will discuss showing the hindquarters. This calming signal is given by horses if they do not want to make contact with others or if they wish to avoid conflict with them. Often they will initially face the stimulus, such as a person or an animal, head on or at an angle, but when the tension increases they turn their hindquarters towards that same provoking or provoked stimulus. A horse who shows his hindquarters demonstrates that he is relaxed and does not want conflict. For that same reason, he will have all four feet planted on the ground, both ears pointed forwards at something entirely different, and he will possibly start to graze (an added calming element). I have mostly seen accompanying head–neck positions of low to mid-high.

The intensity that precedes the horse turning around may vary. In my experience, showing the hindquarters happens mostly from a walk. However, it is also possible for one horse to chase off another, in which case the horse who is chased off will show a couple of paces of walk, trot, or canter before standing still in a position of showing his hindquarters to the aggressor and starting to graze. My assumption is that showing of the hindquarters and the grazing allows the distance put between the two to remain smaller than it would need to have been if the horse had again faced the agitated horse full on.

What stands out is that a horse who shows his hindquarters seems relaxed. (See the photos in the distance increasing signals section in section 3.12.) An example of showing the hindquarters is shown (**Figs 2.109–2.112**).

Showing the hindquarters as a calming signal is something you often see in horses who are housed in busy stables. When they want peace and quiet, they turn their hindquarters towards their stall door. I wish to stress here that the horse in no way means to provoke or threaten to kick. A horse who is threatening to kick looks completely different (see section 3.12). A logical consequence of a horse in a busy stable wanting a little peace and quiet and turning his hindquarters towards the door is that he nods off to sleep. In this situation his head sags down to the horizontal position and he may place one of his hind legs in a rest position. Horses who are outside without shelter in bad weather turn their hindquarters into the wind. They hold their heads lower. In this situation, the turning of the hindquarters is not a calming signal.

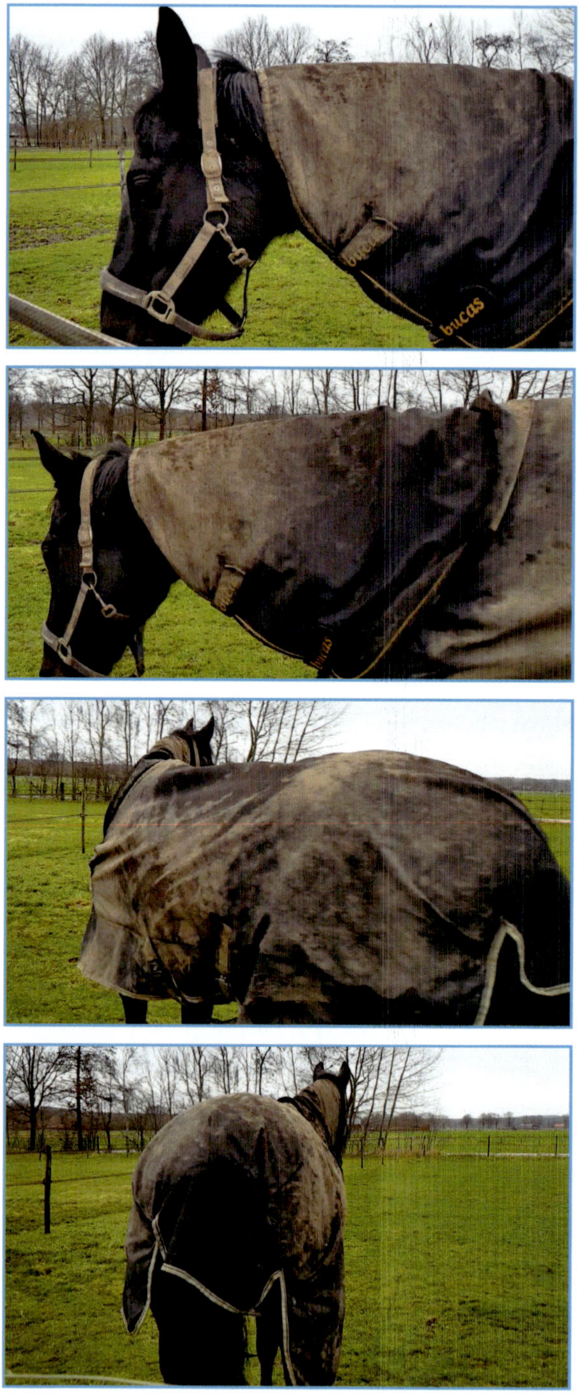

Figs 2.109–2.112 I am filming Prince. He has his answer ready: turning his hindquarters towards me. He does not feel like being in contact with me, but he does not want conflict either. Simply: 'Please Do Not Disturb'. Note that there was no other stimulus to which Prince may have been responding.

2.19 SHOWING THE FLANKS

When a horse shows you his hindquarters, it means he wants neither contact nor conflict at that moment. The horse does not want to disturb or be disturbed. However, instead of his hindquarters, a horse may also turn his flank. This can be either the left or right flank to a person, animal, object, or sound. After the turn, he will stand still, relaxed, with four feet on the ground, both ears pointed forwards or one pointed forwards and the other aimed at the stimulus he is communicating with. His head–neck position is between low and mid-high. There will often be an open space of a few metres between the horse and the object or person to which he is turning his flank. Showing the flank still means 'Do Not Disturb', but there is a definite difference between this and showing the hindquarters. Showing the flank seems to constitute a pause in communication before a possible follow-up move is initiated. After they show their flanks, many horses still take the initiative to meet and investigate the stimulus. However, this usually happens when the stimulus – the person, animal, or object – does not take the initiative to approach the horse and allows the horse to choose his moment of reciprocation. It is especially when people walk firmly towards a horse in a straight line that I see many horses recoil.

A horse who shows his hindquarters or flank usually does not show any other calming signals as he turns. After all, the turning away is one big calming signal in itself. You will, however, often see them show a calming signal after the turn, such as eating, walking away while making a chewing motion, or lowering the head and neck.

This is a recurring pattern when it comes to horses' reactions to unknown objects:

An unknown object lies in the middle of the outdoor arena. A horse is released into the arena. He looks at the object and walks into a corner. There he turns his hindquarters towards the object and starts to graze. After a few minutes (depending on the horse and his experiences in life) he follows the track at a walk towards the letter B or E. He is then parallel with the object, his flank turned towards it. He starts to graze (enabling him to observe the object from a distance). After a few minutes, the horse walks over to the object in a curve in order to examine it.

However, showing the hindquarters or flank is done as a calming signal. So this is done by horses who are careful, polite, and want to calm themselves or the object (**Figs 2.113–2.116**). Horses who want to play or who want to attack or chase away the object (albeit in play), or horses who are used to different kinds of objects, will just approach it in a straight line, without showing the hindquarters or the flank.

NOTE: When your horse is at pasture or in the arena or paddock, you can tell where he wants to go by the direction in which his body is turned.

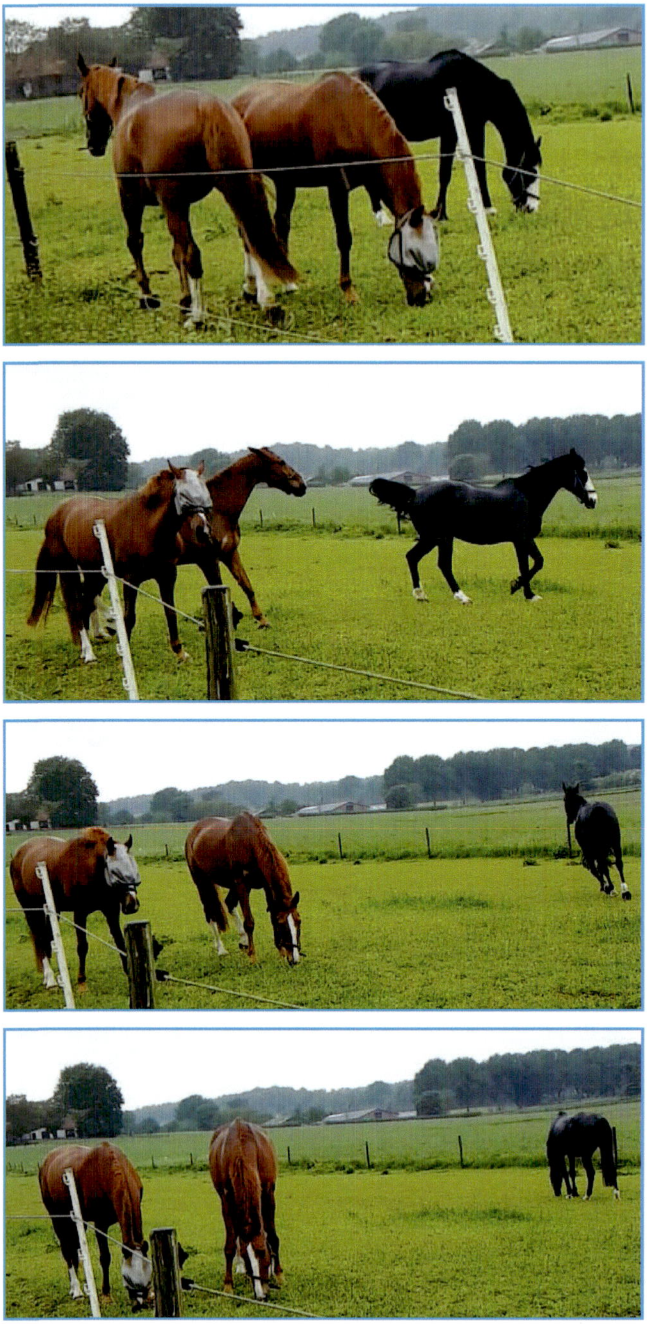

Figs 2.113–2.116 ***Top:*** Oscar, the horse standing on the right, is standing too close to Lorain, the chestnut grazing in the middle. ***Upper middle:*** The chestnut without a fly mask, Vosje, chases Oscar off using a distance increasing signal (see section 3.8). ***Lower middle:*** Oscar moves away. ***Bottom:*** Oscar turns his flanks towards Vosje, and he also starts to eat (two calming signals by means of which he shows that he does not want conflict).

2.20 EATING

At first I found it hard to classify 'eating' as a calming signal. There were a few questions I wanted to look into more thoroughly. Here are two of them:

1 Eating is a necessity of life for the horse, directly linked to his survival and physical wellbeing.

   Just like that of his ancestors, the horse's body is geared towards grazing around the clock. For many domesticated horses, however, this situation no longer applies. There are often large intervals between their feedings, and they do not always get to graze for long periods on pastures with high-quality grass. This can lead to various health problems.[4] One of them is a heightened chance of developing ulcers. The horse's stomach constantly produces gastric acid. When the horse eats, saliva is produced. When, together with the food, the saliva hits the stomach, it neutralises the gastric acid. If a horse does not eat for more than 6 hours and the gastric acid is not neutralised, the chance of ulcers increases.[5] Clearly, many domesticated horses do not meet this criterion, and they will therefore lower their heads to the ground wherever possible to try to find as much grass as they can.

2 Horses are very good at creating feeding opportunities for themselves (even when they are not especially hungry) if this space is given to them (freely or otherwise) by their riders. Think of the horse who snatches a mouthful of hay out of a bale as his rider walks him out of the stable. This is much more a matter of learning by experiment and developing habits than communication.

Despite these two very prevalent and valid reasons, I still could not avoid including eating as a calming signal. So I am attributing it with a communicative function. What has made me decide to do this? Both in horses who met their quota of eating every day and in horses who did not, I saw eating occur within a communicative pattern.

I also saw meaningful variations in the way horses eat and the number of bites they take, variations that fall outside the usual eating pattern. Therefore, I began to study these patterns. I very explicitly counted the number of bites horses took while grazing for 45 minutes as I held them on a rope. I made note of the number of bites between minutes 1–5, minutes 20–25, and minutes 40–45. The horses grazed on the same piece of pasture every time, but the circumstances differed. The weather differed and sometimes there was work being done next to the pasture.

In this study I also observed horses whose tension was increasing. I was able to have a good look at their eating pattern. In general, my findings were:

1 When a horse wants to remove tension and prevent escalation between himself and other stimuli, he will lower his head to the ground to eat (e.g. grass, hay). The way he positions his body in relation to a stimulus provides additional information. If the horse has turned his flank to the

stimulus (a supplementary calming signal), then he is taking a break. He watches the stimulus as he eats, and may or may not choose to approach it. If the horse is standing with his hindquarters facing the stimulus and eating, he is giving a stronger signal that he does not want to interact with the stimulus. He has ended the communication (for a longer time). If the horse faces the stimulus, he will approach it after a moment.

2 Chewing and eating cause a reduction in tension. If a horse cannot eat because he is in a place where there is no food available, you will often see him sniffing the ground and stirring up the ground with his nose. In this context this is not displacement behaviour (see section 2.23), but an attempt to find a blade of grass.

3 The higher the tension, the higher the bite frequency. The horse takes more bites than he would if he were relaxed. The bite technique may also be different. Because of the tension, the horse may open his mouth a little wider before he takes a bite, or he might lift his upper lip a little and bare his upper teeth a bit more when he bites.

4 If the tension rises even further, then the horse is no longer able to eat. He takes a bite but no longer chews, finally letting the food fall from his mouth and ceasing to eat altogether.

EATING TOGETHER CONNECTS

Horses naturally eat in a herd, so eating grass is something they naturally do together. It is a social activity. My view is that this is a crucial difference between horses and their riders. Riders feel a connection with their horse when they are riding. I think horses feel connected to others when they are eating together. I think a horse is more likely to become attached to his rider or handler when he or she hand walks him, allowing him to eat along the way, than when riding.

Eating grass is often seen as a bad habit by riders and handlers. Riders complain that their horse stops at every tuft of grass to take a bite, even when the rider does not want him to. However, I see allowing the horse to eat as a good tool to calm him down (**Figs 2.117, 2.118**). When he has calmed down, which is discernible from the way he eats, then move on. It may be that in the beginning there is a period in which your horse wants to eat grass wherever he goes. In my experience, when you start hand walking the horse more often and allowing him to eat along the way, he will come with you much more easily. You can also work on a word that invites the horse to eat and one that tells him it is time to stop eating and you are moving on.

However, a horse who does not want to eat cannot be forced to eat. He feels tense. In that case the situation will have to be changed in such a way that the horse's tension drops. There may of course also be an underlying disease or ailment at the root of it, necessitating an appointment with a veterinarian dentist.

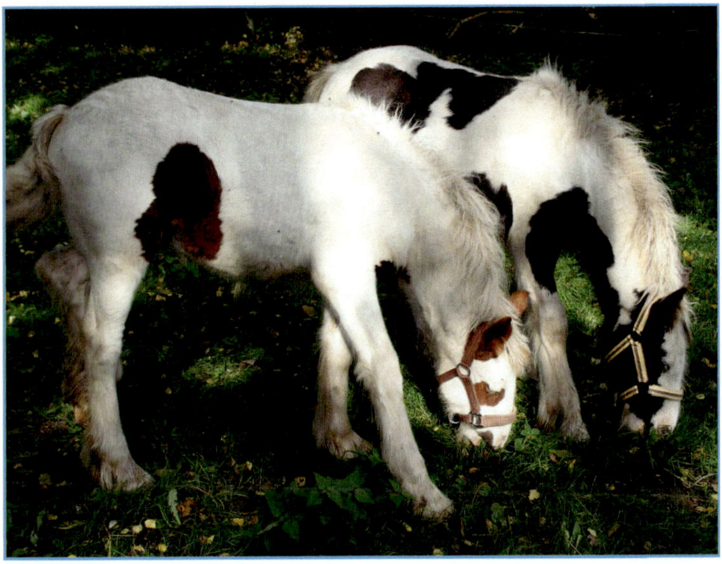

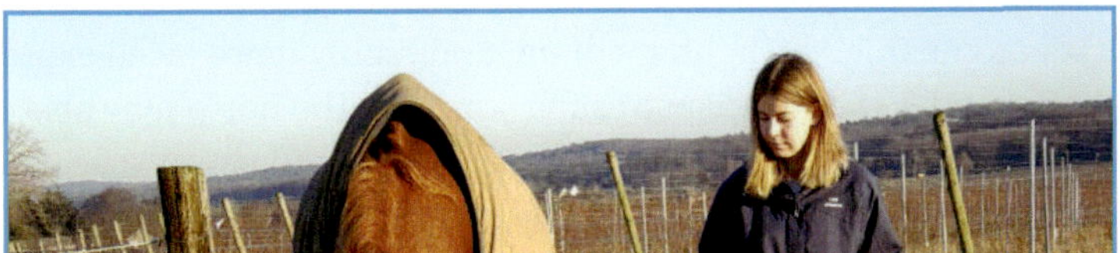

Figs 2.117, 2.118 Eating as a means of calming and bonding.

2.21 IMMOBILITY AND SLOWING DOWN

There are three types of immobility a horse can demonstrate:

1 Immobility in response to a stimulus.
2 Immobility in response to high tension: a freeze.
3 Immobility and slowing down as a calming signal.

IMMOBILITY AFTER A LIGHT AND STRONG STIMULUS

A horse shows this type of immobility as a direct result of a stimulus (**Fig. 2.119**). The horse stops whatever he is doing to literally stop and stare. The horse lifts his head to a mid-high to high position. His ears are pointed in the direction of the stimulus he wants to identify. He uses his senses to determine what he is experiencing. The degree to which the horse recognises and is able to handle the stimulus determines the level of tension. If the new stimulus is subtle and the horse recognises and understands it, then there is a moment of light tension, after which the horse can resume whatever he was doing before the stimulus arrived.

If the stimulus is less recognisable to the horse, then the moment in which he stands still is accompanied by light, medium, and highly tense facial expressions (see sections 3.3 and 3.4). In response to the stimulus, the horse may also show calming signals or mild intentions to fight or flee by moving away a few paces. In summary, the immobility is not a calming signal in itself, it is a physical reaction to a stimulus. However, the horse may show calming signals in response to this stimulus.

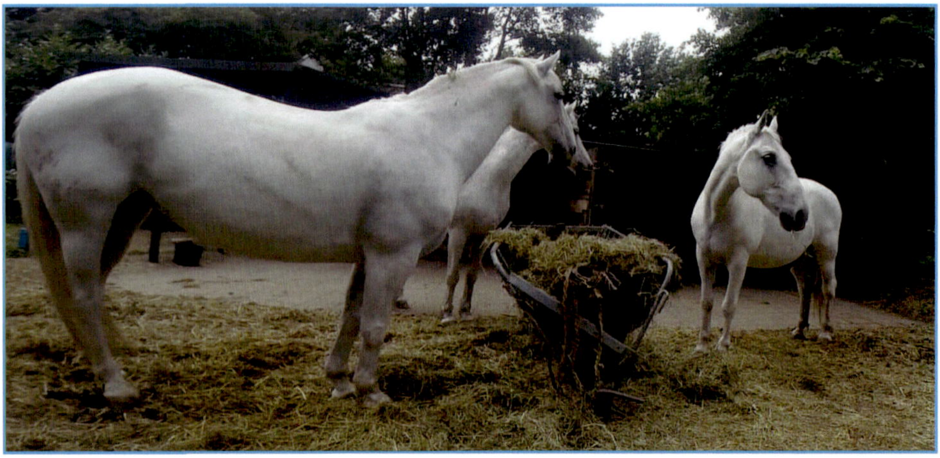

Fig. 2.119 These Lipizzaners are eating. All of a sudden, they hear a sound. They raise their heads to the mid-high position, stand stock still, and stop chewing the hay. After 3 seconds of assessing the sound, it is deemed safe and they start eating again.

IMMOBILITY IN CASE OF HIGH TENSION: A FREEZE

If the level of tension in response to a new stimulus is very high, immobility becomes a kind of stiffening: a freeze. The horse lifts his head high, shows facial features that are associated with high tension, and all the muscles in his body are tensed. This is not a calming signal, but a direct physical reaction to danger. During a freeze, there are no longer any calming signals or displacement activities. This is discussed further in Chapter 3.

IMMOBILITY AND SLOWING DOWN AS CALMING SIGNALS

I often see immobility and calming down as calming signals in an interaction between horses, between horses and other animals, or between horses and some other stimulus. Within the interaction there is a disruptive element, leading one of the horses to use standing still and slowing down as a calming signal. This may happen, for example, when a horse is curious about an object and wants to approach it, but does so carefully. He walks very slowly (slowed down), stops from time to time, then stands still, and finally moves again, very slowly. When a horse shows this behaviour pattern, you will also often see other calming signals, such as curving, or see-saw or sustained lowering, or a head or neck turn.

Immobility and slowing down also occur when a horse wants to approach, for example, an object, horse, or other animal that is already being shielded by another horse. For the sake of convenience, let us call that horse the protector. By slowly approaching the coveted object – the water trough, for instance, or another horse – and stopping and standing immobile every once in a while, the horse tries to appease the protector and ensure the success of his action. Whether he does or not depends on the object and the value the protector attributes to it. When horses use immobility as a calming signal, the muscles are not tensed beyond what is needed to stay in position. This is fundamentally different from a freeze, during which all the muscles are tensed. All head–neck positions are possible during immobility and slowing down as calming signals, and other calming signals may also be shown.

2.22 SUMMARY: CALMING SIGNALS

- Calming signals are meant to achieve or maintain good social relations, to be polite, and to avoid conflict.
- Calming signals calm both the other horse and the horse himself.
- If calming signals work, they allow the horse to stay in that situation.
- All calming signals can be given as single signals. After giving one or two, the horse usually becomes relaxed again, just as he was before the signal.
- It is also possible for multiple signals to be given. These can be given simultaneously or sequentially. After giving a few signals, the horse may return to a relaxed state. However, the more calming signals are given, and the faster they succeed one another, the more the horse's tension rises.
- Calming signals are also given when a horse is recovering from a big shock or tension. The calming signals are the last step to relaxation.

2.23 ALTERNATING DISPLACEMENT BEHAVIOUR AND CALMING SIGNALS

You are standing at a bus stop, waiting for your bus. A young guy walks up and stands next to you. You give him a nod and say, 'Hello'. He does not respond. He does not return your greeting and moves to stand in front of you, looking you in the eye. You turn away from him a little and start to study the bus schedule, posted nearby, even though you already know that your bus will arrive in 5 minutes.

In this scenario, the basic situation is that you are relaxed as you stand at the bus stop. The young man's arrival is the stimulus that makes you give calming signals: nodding and saying hello. The young man does not respond with a calming signal, such as a return greeting or looking away a little. He keeps facing you and maintains eye contact. Maybe you wanted to walk away from him, displaying flight behaviour, but then you would have missed your bus. Maybe you wanted to tell him to stop staring at you, thus proactively changing the situation (a fight response). But you do neither. Instead you release some of the built-up tension by showing entirely different behaviour (called displacement behaviour) that does not provoke the other. This is not a derivative or weaker form of walking away or fighting, but a behaviour from an entirely different category of behaviours: reading the bus schedule, even though you never intended to do that.

I think displacement activities are intended to release tension, to focus on something else because you cannot display the behaviour you really want to display. This may be because you do not want confrontation or escalation, are being impeded, or because it is not appropriate in your particular social context. Displacement activities are not intensified forms of behaviour that were shown before that moment. They are new behaviours that turn the attention on oneself and do not provoke the other person. Here are some examples of displacement activities humans use: scratching our head, fussing with clothes or buttons, reading messages on our phone, picking at the table's edge.

Displacement activities can also be regular behaviours. After all, you can also scratch your head when you have an itch, or fuss with a button on your blouse after it has come undone. But displacement behaviours can also be recognised because they can be part of a sequence of behaviours. There is a stimulus that stimulates, for instance, a horse to respond. The horse gives calming signals, but the calming signals do not cause the situation to change. The tension remains. The horse shows displacement behaviours to release the internal tension. While showing a displacement activity the horse focuses solely on the activity and his attention is not on the environment.

An example. A horse is in a small paddock. Some children walk up and they start to lean over the fence. They face the horse fully. The horse shows calming signals. He turns his head away and blinks. He does this more than once. He then starts to extensively rub his head along his foreleg (displacement behaviour). He chews for a moment, then walks away.

Displacement activities can occur in two ways in communication sequences:

1. Displacement behaviour succeeds the calming signals if there is rising tension in the horse. This may be a smooth step upwards in the communication sequence if the horse's tension rises gradually. It may also be the case that the displacement activities and calming signals alternate a bit for a period. This happens when a stimulus causes light tension in the horse, but this tension does not develop into either higher tension or relaxation.
2. The horse is very tense, for example due to a startle response. When the tension starts to decrease, the horse shows displacement behaviour and then calming signals on the way to relaxation (this is discussed further in section 3.20).

DISPLACEMENT ACTIVITIES ARE SKIPPED

When do you not see displacement behaviours after calming signals in a behaviour sequence?

1. When the horse's tension rises so quickly that after giving the calming signals, he skips the displacement activities and goes straight to stress signals.
2. When the horse is using stereotyped behaviour, such as weaving, for example. A stereotyped behaviour is a movement that is made repeatedly without pause. The horse seems self-absorbed while doing it. Stereotyped behaviour looks like pointless behaviour to people, but it does serve a purpose as a coping mechanism.[6]
3. When the external stimulus lessens or goes away entirely, the calming signals have helped the horse to lower his light internal tension. Displacement behaviour is not activated. This situation is described in the previous section.

A communication pattern that includes calming signals and displacement behaviour, after which the tension decreases, is shown in section 2.24.

2.24 COMMUNICATION LADDER: DISPLACEMENT BEHAVIOUR

Ladder 2.2

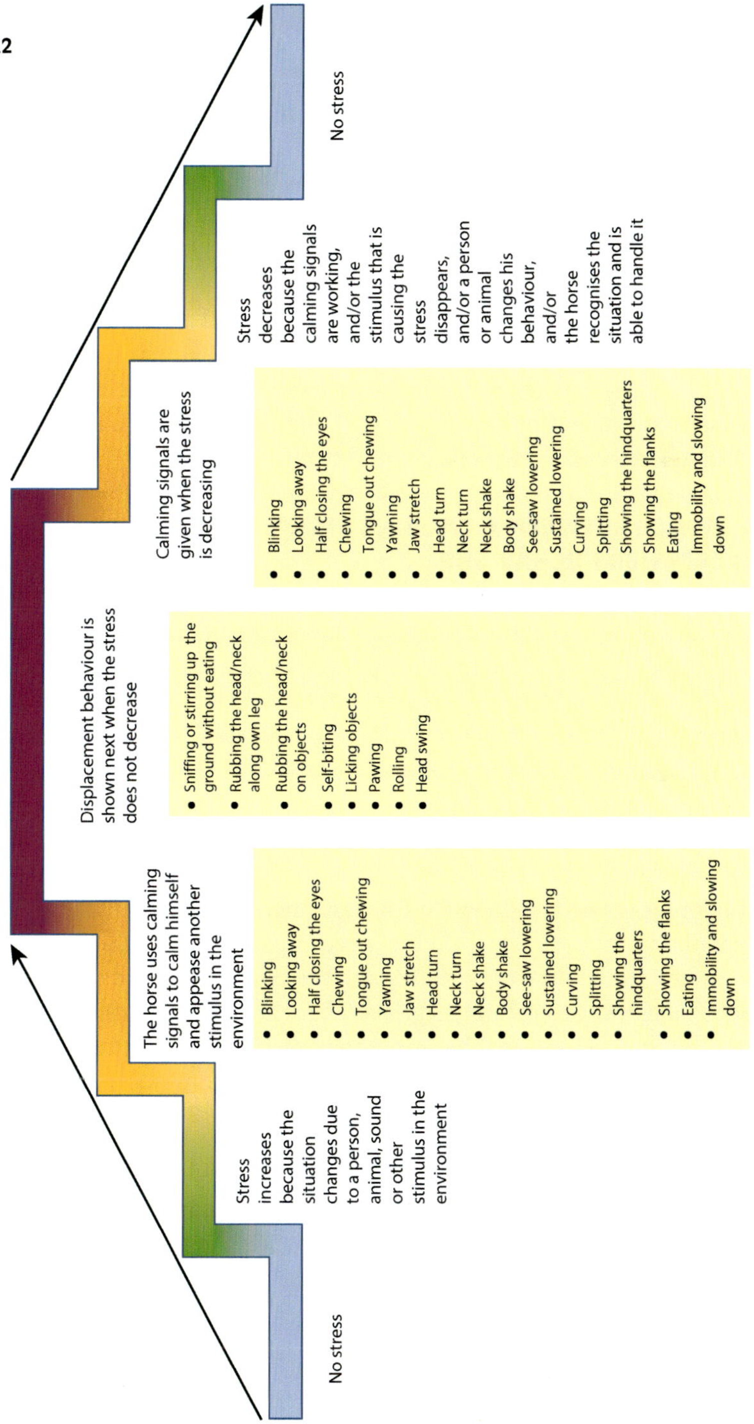

2.25 FACES AND BEHAVIOURS

Displacement behaviours can follow and alternate with every calming signal. They can be shown from every head–neck position and afterwards the horse can also come back to every possible head–neck position. During displacement activities, the horse's mouth is usually active and an integral part of the behaviour in question, such as licking, biting, or sniffing the ground.

The horse can show displacement behaviours with a face that carries light, medium, or high tension, according to the level of tension the horse is feeling at that moment. The facial features of a horse who is feeling rising tension are discussed in Chapter 3, which is all about tension.

All displacement behaviours also have a self-contained biological function. The horse can sniff the ground and stir it up in order to smell. He can grind and bite because of an itch. He can lick to taste. It is up to the handler to tell the difference between when the horse is performing these behaviours to fulfil a biological function and when they are part of a communicative sequence.

THE DIFFERENCE BETWEEN A CALMING SIGNAL AND DISPLACEMENT BEHAVIOUR

During my research, I have seen a lot of body signals that were given in a single long sequence, without breaks in between, like a string of pearls. For instance, you will see a horse blink, chew, tongue out chew, yawn, and do a jaw stretch in an effortless progression. With those cases, I did not feel that the displacement activities were really part of an entirely different behaviour system. However, I do feel this when it comes to the displacement behaviours I discuss in this chapter. To me, these behaviours are of a different character from the movements shown before. They are also a little bigger in terms of physical activity. I also think that with these displacement activities, the horse seems to disconnect from his environment for longer in order to become one with the movement. My categorisation of displacement behaviours differs from that of scientists. For example, scientists label yawning, the jaw stretch, the neck shake, and the body shake as displacement behaviours. I label these as calming signals. These are the displacement behaviours that I have seen in my study, that have met my criterion of occurring at least 35 times, and that I have chosen to mention or discuss more extensively.

2.26 DISPLACEMENT ACTIVITIES

Some examples of displacement activities are shown in **Figs 2.120–2.125**.

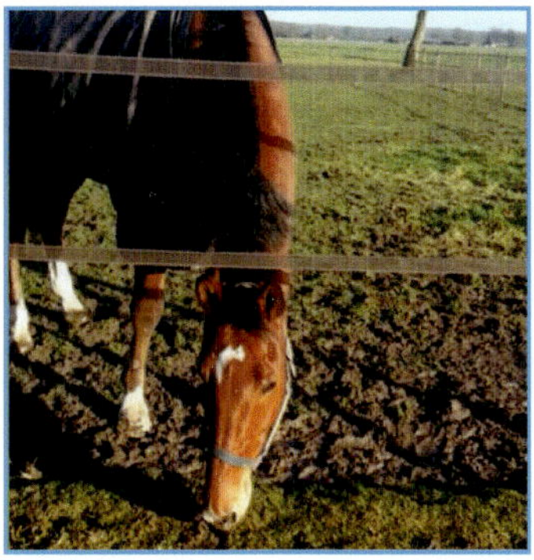

Fig. 2.120 Sniffing or stirring up the ground without eating.

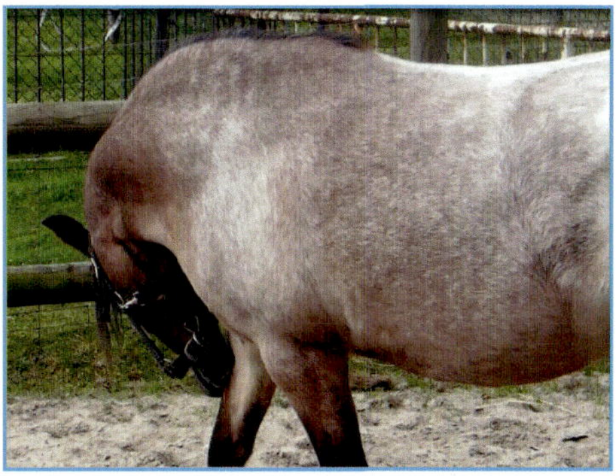

Fig. 2.121 Self-biting.

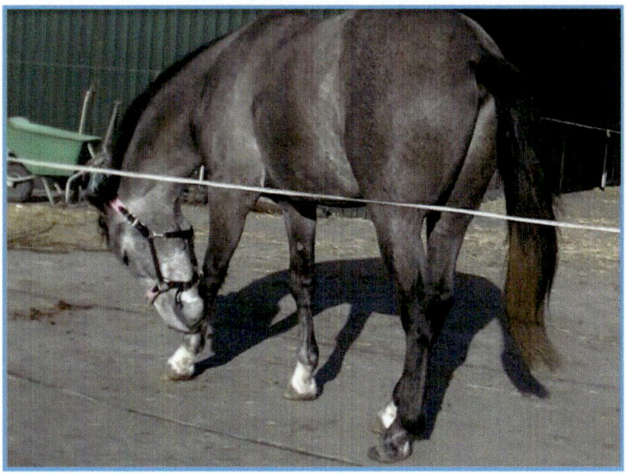

Fig. 2.122 Rubbing the head along own leg.

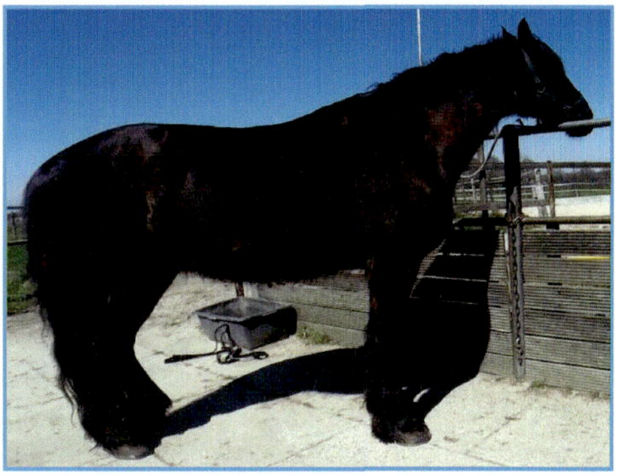

Fig. 2.123 Rubbing the head or neck on objects.

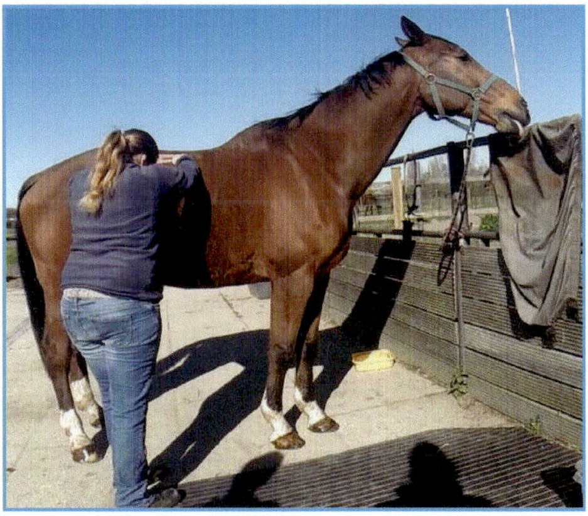

Fig. 2.124 Licking objects.

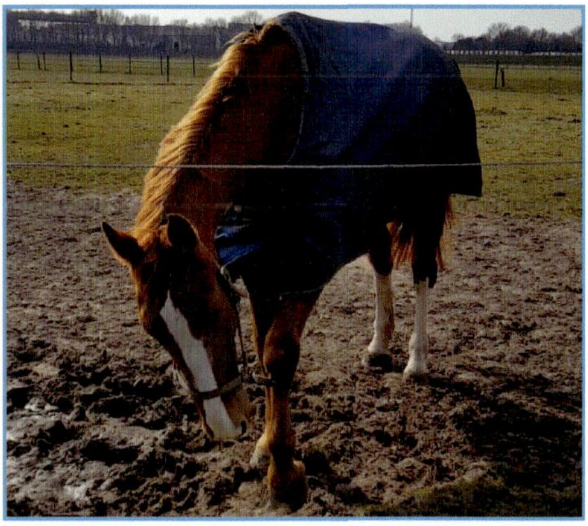

Fig. 2.125 Pawing (scraping the foreleg on the ground).

2.27 ROLLING

When rolling is not a displacement behaviour, horses take their time over it. They lower their neck and often sniff the ground extensively to find the best place in which to roll. They often walk in small circles while doing this. They paw the ground a number of times and slowly lower themselves onto their forelegs. They roll and move a number of times on one side and sometimes rub their head and neck across the ground. It is also possible for them to roll from one side, past their tipping point, to their other side. After rolling, the horse does a full body shake and calmly walks away.

Rolling as displacement behaviour is characterised by haste (**Figs 2.126–2.131**). First, the horse already feels light tension, so he walks more quickly to the place where he is going to roll. It is also possible for a horse to approach the rolling spot at a slow trot. There is usually no extensive search for a good spot. The horse lowers his head and immediately lowers himself onto his forelegs in order to roll. He often rolls once on one side, maybe tipping over once, and gets up again. He trots or canters away, possibly showing a head swing, or stands still with a very high head–neck position.

The pawing is skipped, or the horse does only one or two paws instead of the usual three to four. In comparison with rolling for the sake of grooming, this roll lasts for a much shorter time. It also has fewer rolling motions. After a grooming roll, the horse does a full body shake. This is less prevalent after rolling as displacement behaviour. In this situation, the horse sometimes only does a neck shake. After the shake, the horse shows heightened physical activity as it moves on, maybe in the form of trotting or cantering away or bucking. If the horse releases more tension, he will show more calming signals and displacement behaviour.

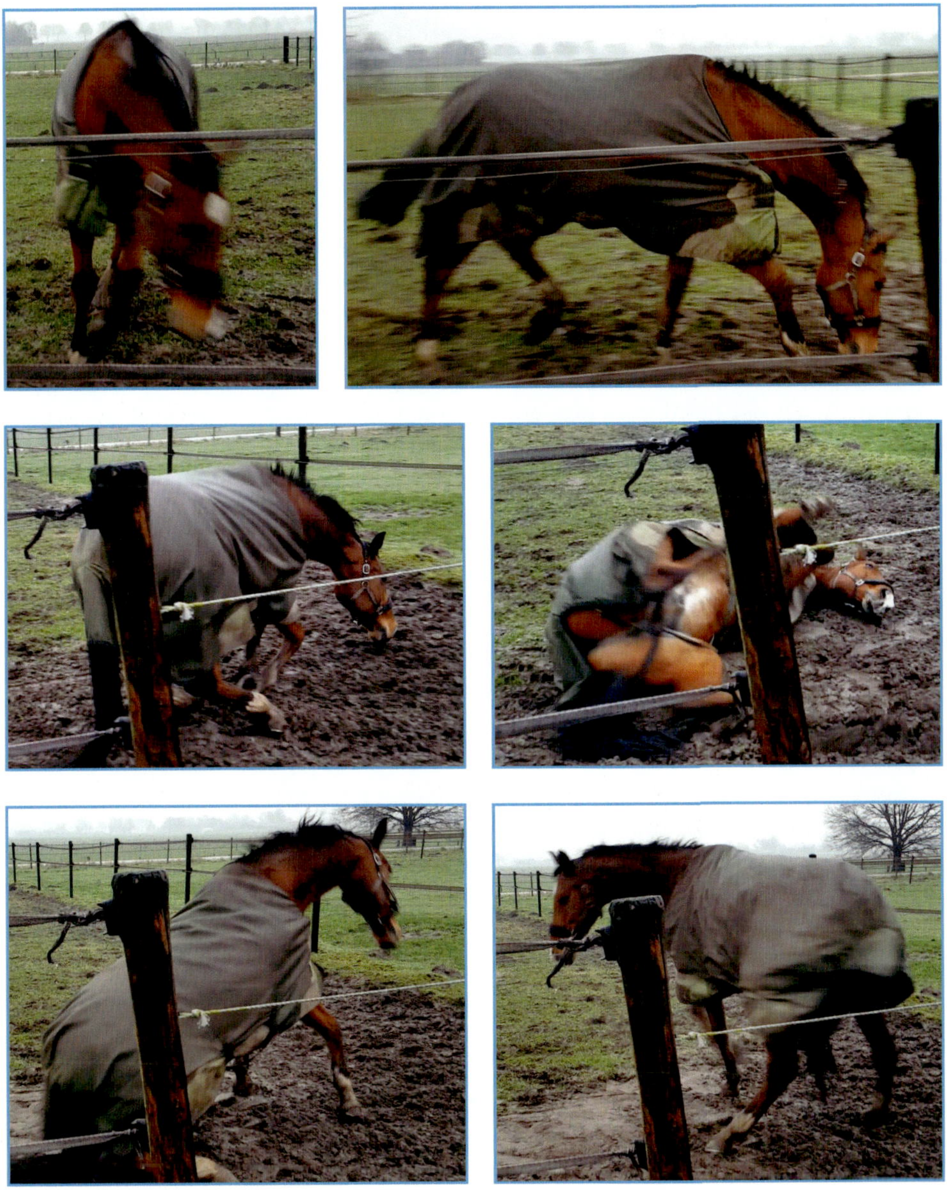

Figs 2.126–2.131 These photos show rolling as displacement behaviour. The horse does two entire rolling cycles in 26 seconds. After this first roll, the horse did another roll straight away. You can see the start of this in the last photo.

2.28 HEAD SWING

A head swing is characterised by the horse doing a swaying, rotating motion with his whole head.

In this swing, the horse's head may be completely horizontal at one point. The neck turns with the head swing. In my research, I have seen a head swing done from a standstill, a walk, a trot, and a canter. After a head swing, the horse can carry on in all gaits. During a head swing, the tail may be carried and swished (**Figs 2.132, 2.133**).

The head swing is one of the signals that occurs in multiple places on the communication ladder. This is because a head swing has many different levels of intensity. If a horse performs a head swing under light tension or because of a weak internal motivation, the resulting head swing is less powerful, often consisting only of an initial mobilisation and a light swing sideways with the head. If a horse performs a head swing under high tension or because of a strong internal motivation, then the resulting head and neck swing is powerful and pronounced. I have seen a head swing as the following:

- As displacement behaviour. Here you will see a head swing after the horse has given a number of calming signals. The horse's tension remains, and he cannot display the behaviour he wishes to display. In this situation, the head swing is a displacement behaviour that allows his tension to decrease. After doing this head swing, and possibly showing some other mild displacement activities such as pawing, rubbing the head along the foreleg, or grooming by self-biting, the tension has lowered, and the horse may show some calming signals, or skip these and return to his basic state of relaxation.
- If the horse feels more tension and this is not ebbing, a more powerful head swing may also be shown in combination with other behaviours that are more physically energetic, such as rolling, bucking, and trotting away. If a head swing is used as a tension releaser, you will see that horse focus only on himself, not on someone else. With the type of head swing described next, however, you will see the horse focus on another.
- A head swing may also be a harbinger of a desire to drive others away. This can be horses, people, dogs, or other objects. This can happen on the basis of a weak or strong motivation, which is then reflected in the strength or weakness of the head swing. With a weak motivation the associated movement patterns are standing still and walking, and with a stronger motivation, trotting and cantering. When a head swing is used to drive others away, immediately before or right after the head swing you will see the horse focus his total attention on the one he wants to chase away.
- A head swing can also be a part of play.
- A head swing may also be a reaction to pain. The horse may experience a pain stimulus in the mouth, perhaps due to dental pain or the rider yanking on the bit too hard.

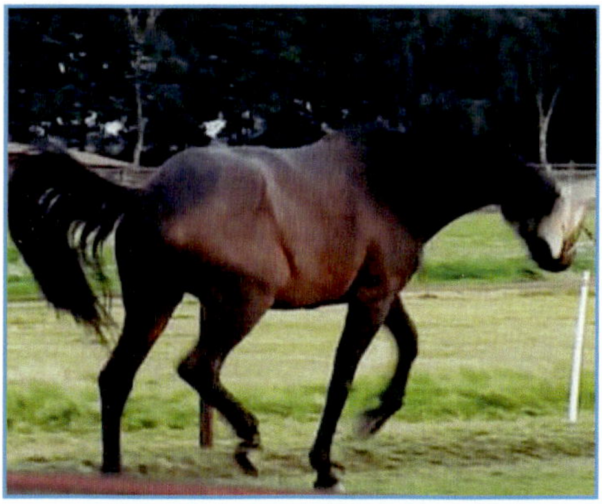

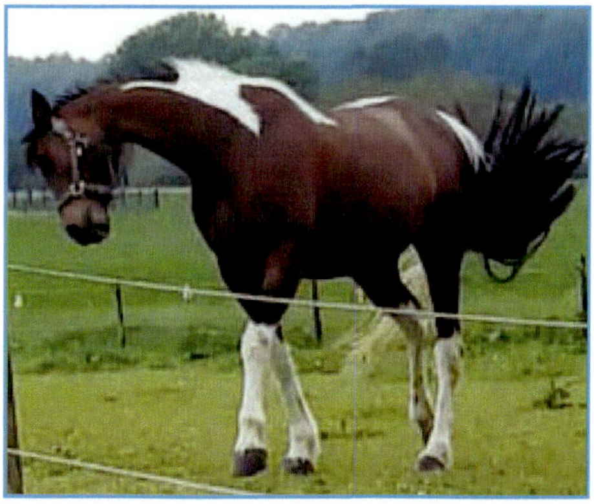

Figs 2.132, 2.133 Horses demonstrating head swinging.

THE MORE RESTRICTION, THE MORE DISPLACEMENT BEHAVIOUR

At home, while travelling, or in unknown places, the domesticated horse is often restricted in his freedom of movement. He is tied up for grooming and, while he is being saddled, has to wait in his stall or in a trailer or is confined in a temporary box at a competition. From a human practical perspective this tying and locking up is understandable. The horse is safe and the handler has his hands free to do other things. However, it is sensible to wonder if the horse can actually handle this situation, being alone in a box or trailer, being without other horses, or being in a place full of unfamiliar sights, sounds, and smells. I have seen many horses who showed calming signals and displacement behaviour especially when they were tied up or locked in a trailer, stall, or unfamiliar box at a competition. Some horses were so tense that they even showed stress signals and distance increasing signals.

Horses who were locked in a stall, who wanted to get out but could not, displayed displacement behaviours such as pawing, licking objects (like walls and doors), or rubbing their head along their leg, or the side of an opened shutter. Horses who were tied up on a rope and who did not want to stand still would often paw, rub their head on a foreleg, or bite their chest or foreleg, or both.

There were also horses who, from a confined position, showed stereotyped behaviours. These stereotyped behaviours come directly on the heels of a calming signal or displacement behaviour. It may also be that the confined horse was showing weakened fight or flight signals.

The owners responded differently to the stereotyped and displacement behaviours. A percentage of them did not notice. A percentage responded by stroking or speaking comfortingly to their horse.

Horses I saw who displayed stereotyped behaviours were not punished by their owners or prevented from doing them. And a good thing too; research shows that this is a coping mechanism for a horse that allows him to better deal with a situation. Punishment or preventing the horse from executing the behaviour leads to higher stress levels.[6]

2.29 EXAMPLE OF CALMING SIGNALS AND DISPLACEMENT BEHAVIOUR

The series of eight photos below are of a horse who is showing several calming signals and a displacement behaviour (**Figs 2.134–2.141**).

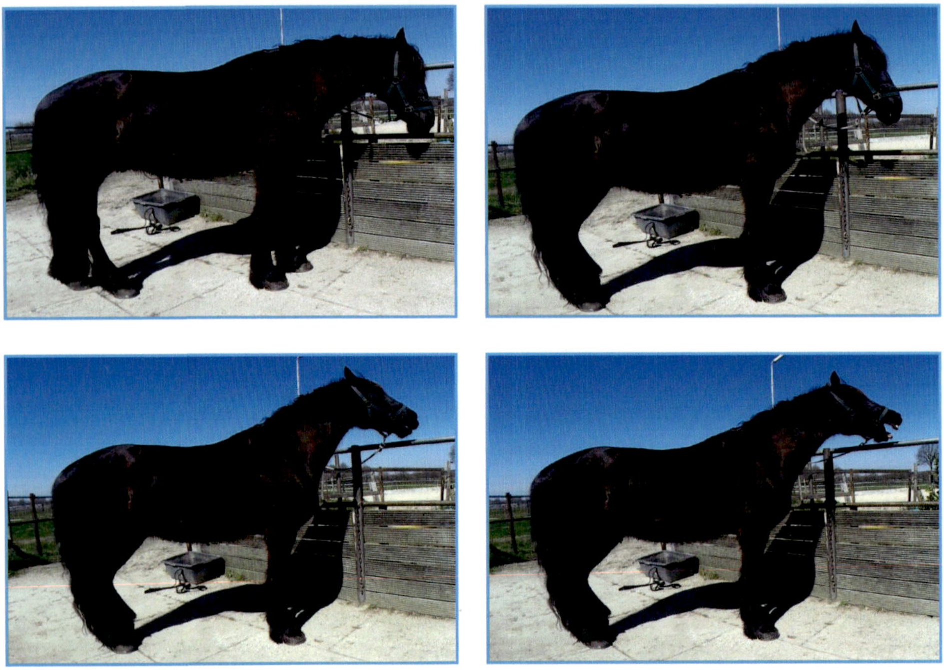

Figs 2.134–2.141 Itske is tied up, waiting for the saddle maker. The goal is to find a saddle that fits. The wait is rather long, however. Itske shows several calming signals. The photos show Itske waiting, chewing, doing a jaw stretch, yawning, rubbing his chin on a pole (displacement behaviour), yawning several more times (five times in the video footage), tongue out chewing, and finally patiently waiting again. What is not shown in the photos, but is visible on the video footage, is the fact that in between the photos, Itske chews and also does a few see-saw lowerings. The time interval between the photos is 90 seconds.

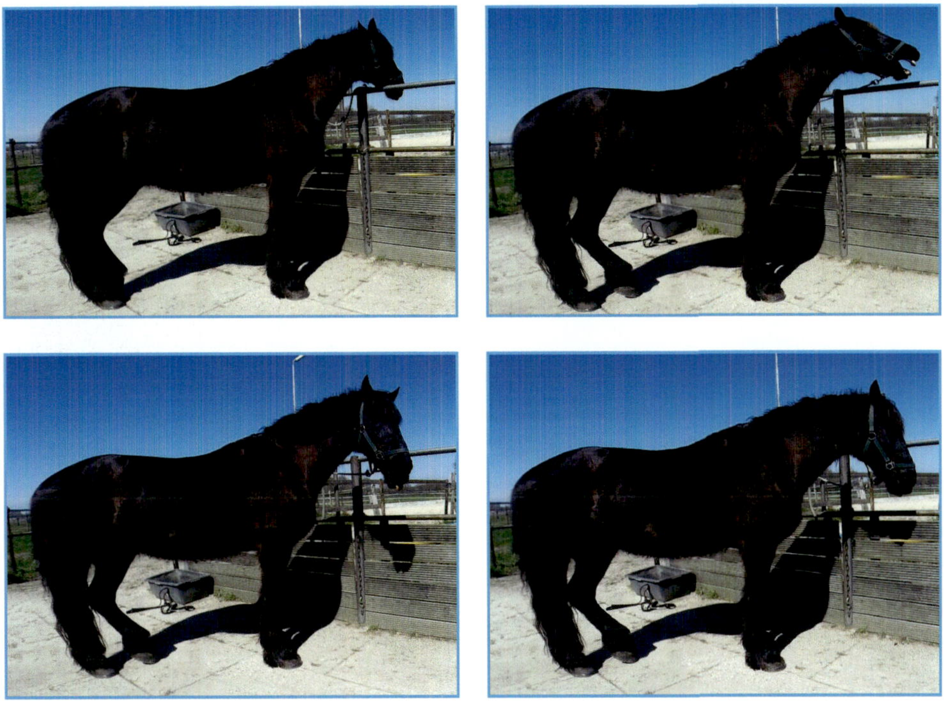

Figs 2.134–2.141 *(Continued)*

2.30 SUMMARY: DISPLACEMENT BEHAVIOUR

- Displacement behaviour is intended to let the horse release tension. While showing the displacement behaviour, they disconnect from the situation and communication with others.
- Displacement behaviour occurs within a communication pattern and is preceded by multiple simultaneous or consecutive calming signals.
- Displacement behaviour can result in two outcomes:
  1. The tension lessens and calming signals are given, after which the tensions ebbs further.
  2. The tension increases. The horse gives more stress signals, possibly distance increasing signals or weakened forms of these.
- When there is increasing tension, calming signals transition into displacement behaviour. However, if the increasing tension suddenly peaks, the horse skips displacement behaviour and goes straight to giving stress signals.
- As a coping mechanism, the horse may also follow calming signals with stereotyped behaviour instead of displacement behaviour.
- Calming signals and displacement activities allow the horse to get through a situation. If the horse shows stress signals, then his body is readying itself to proactively leave or change the situation.

2.31 REFERENCES

1 Neugebauer GM, Neugebauer JK (2011) *Het gedrag van paarden beter begrijpen*. Eugen Ulmer KG, Stuttgart, p. 96.
2 McBane S (2012) *Horse Senses*. Manson Publishing Ltd, London, p. 77.
3 McBane S (2012) *Horse Senses*. Manson Publishing Ltd, London, p. 33.
4 Davidson N, Harris P (2003) Nutrition and welfare. In: *The Welfare of Horses*. (ed. N Waran) Kluwer Academic Publishers, Dordrecht, pp. 45–76.
5 Sykes BW, Hewetson M, Hepburn RJ *et al.* (2015) European College of Equine Internal Medicine Consensus Statement – Equine Gastric Ulcer Syndrome in Adult Horses. *J Vet Intern Med* **29(5):**1288–1299. https://www.ncbi.nlm.nih.gov/pmc/articles/PMC4858038
6 Cooper J, McGreevy P (2003) Stereotypic behaviour in the stabled horse: causes, effects and prevention without compromising horse welfare. In: *The Welfare of Horses*. (ed. N Waran) Kluwer Academic Publishers, Dordrecht, pp. 99–124.

3 *Tension shimmers through calming signals*

A BROOM falling over, a dog barking, a paddock the horse does not like but has to stay in, the fear the horse feels when he has to leave his stablemates, pain from a lash of the whip, a training programme that is too demanding, being too hot or cold: tension comes in all shapes and sizes in the life of a domesticated horse. I distinguish below between two types of tension:

1 **Acute stress:** the horse experiences a single moment of stress from which he recovers. Depending on the severity of the shock, tension, or pain, and the horse's own recovery rate, this recovery can take more or less time. More than one moment of acute stress followed by recovery can occur within a certain time frame.
2 **Prolonged (chronic) stress:** the horse finds himself in a situation that causes him stress for a longer period in which no recovery takes place. This often happens if environmental factors continually cause the horse stress, or if there are so many moments of acute tension that the horse has no opportunity to recover and find a mentally and physically healthy balance. This can happen, for example, if the horse is taken to a competition that lasts for several days when he is not yet ready for it, or if he is moved to a new home and takes days, weeks, or months to get used to the new home.

Both types of tension commence the same way with the body preparing to jump into action. Generally, this happens as follows:

Through the amygdala, the fear centre of the brain, the pituitary gland, the hypothalamus sends a signal to the adrenal glands, telling them to secrete catecholamines. Catecholamines include the hormones adrenaline and noradrenaline. These hormones elevate the horse's blood glucose level and raise his blood pressure and heart rate. Blood is pumped through the horse's body faster to allow nutrients to reach his muscles more quickly. The horse's reflexes are faster and his tempo is higher. His breathing also becomes shallower. His body prepares for injury and his immune system is boosted. A few minutes after the hypothalamus has instructed the adrenal glands to secrete catecholamines, another signal is sent to the adrenal glands, this time to secrete glucocorticoids. These include, among others, the hormone cortisol. The role of glucocorticoids is to regulate the catecholamines, thus preventing exhaustion of the body. In this way, the hormone and glucose levels can be regulated again, allowing the body to recover from the shock. They do, however, provide enough energy for the body to continue to function in tense circumstances. For example, a zebra that is under attack from a lion. The amygdala recognises the life-threatening situation and adrenaline and noradrenaline are secreted by the adrenaline glands. This is the booster, and the zebra starts running for his life. If the zebra has not been eaten by the lion in the first seconds or minutes, the body secretes cortisol. This enables the zebra to continue fleeing from the lion for a longer stretch. Cortisol tells the body not to sleep or eat. If the zebra survives and is not eaten by the lion, the body can recover from the tension. A very useful system! Problems arise, however, if a horse is placed in a situation in which he experiences so many moments of acute stress that no regulation and recovery can take place and there is a constantly fluctuating secretion of catecholamines and glucocorticoids. The continuous secretion of cortisol then becomes a cause of health problems for the horse. For example:

- Lacking a feeling of homeostasis: no balanced sense of wellbeing.[1]
- Possibly a more difficult cooperation with his handlers and riders.
- Reduced functioning of the hippocampus: cell activity decreases, there are fewer synapses, and there is less information transferral, which leads to reduced cognitive learning capacity, a reduced ability to solve problems, and reduced memory capacity.[2–4]
- The threshold at which the horse responds fearfully lowers. The horse is startled more quickly and more often, now in addition by things that never used to startle him.[2,5]
- Increased risk of stereotyped behaviours.[6]
- Increased risk of developing injurious behaviours such as self-mutilation and increased aggression.[7]
- Increased risk of developing lethargy and depression.[3,8] This happens because in time the adrenal glands become exhausted.
- Reduced fertility.[9]
- Gastric disorders and damage.[7]
- Weakening of the immune system, which may lead to poorer health.[2,9]

NEW STIMULI NECESSARY FOR CELL PRODUCTION

Considering all these disadvantages, you can appreciate that it is important to keep assessing if a certain training scheme suits the horse and if he understands what he sees and can handle the situation. For this, balance is the magic word. Every mammal, including humans, horses, and dogs, needs stimuli to keep generating cell renewal in the brain, to become and remain mentally fit. Performing suitable physical exercises that the horse's body and mind can handle, stimulating the senses, and facing mental challenges is very important for stimulating a horse; it will also help maintain the horse's joy of life and not let it descend into a life of boredom and depression. Therefore, a horse needs to regularly receive new stimuli, but not be overstimulated. You want the horse to be attentive, interested, and internally motivated, but you do not want the tension to rise to such a degree that the horse cannot handle it any more. Tips for this are provided in section 5.3.

3.1 TENSION RISES DUE TO INCREASING STIMULUS INTENSITY

A horse is at pasture. Suddenly, the sound of a power drill comes from a house nearby. The horse shows calming signals and displacement activities.

The situation can then develop in this way:

1 The calming signals and displacement behaviours calm the horse down. He shows a few more calming signals and the tension wanes (see **Ladder 2.2**). OR

2 The calming signals and displacement behaviour do not help the horse. The situation remains unchanged and the horse's tension rises. In addition to the calming signals and displacement behaviour, the horse shows stress signals.

In the communication ladder below (**3.1**), the horse's tension can come back down when the stimulus ceases or when the horse is moved (or is able to move himself) further away from the stimulus, to a distance at which he can handle it. Or, after a longer time frame in which his tension falls to light tension, the horse recognises the situation and/or stimulus and is able to handle it.

The farrier is tending to Vosje, who is tied up near his stall and has hay to eat. He has done one foreleg and is now moving to Vosje's hind leg. Vosje becomes a bit more restless. He stops eating and lifts his head higher. His nostrils go from long and relaxed to round, and his eyes also become rounder. The farrier trims the hoof on the left hind leg. Vosje defecates. The farrier walks back to the left hind leg, wanting to continue. I call a break.

This scenario shows that rising tension does not need to be accompanied by a lot of physical activity. Horses who are tied up, standing still (horses who have learned that it is impossible for them to flee or fight like this) or in a stall, can still build up a lot of tension on the inside. They just express it in a less obvious way. They may turn and walk a little while attached to the rope. This does not indicate to the handler that there is any need to help the horse. However, this horse could use some help. When in doubt, look at the body posture and facial features of the horse. An overview of the body posture and facial features can be found in section 3.3.

3.2 COMMUNICATION LADDER: STRESS SIGNALS

Ladder 3.1

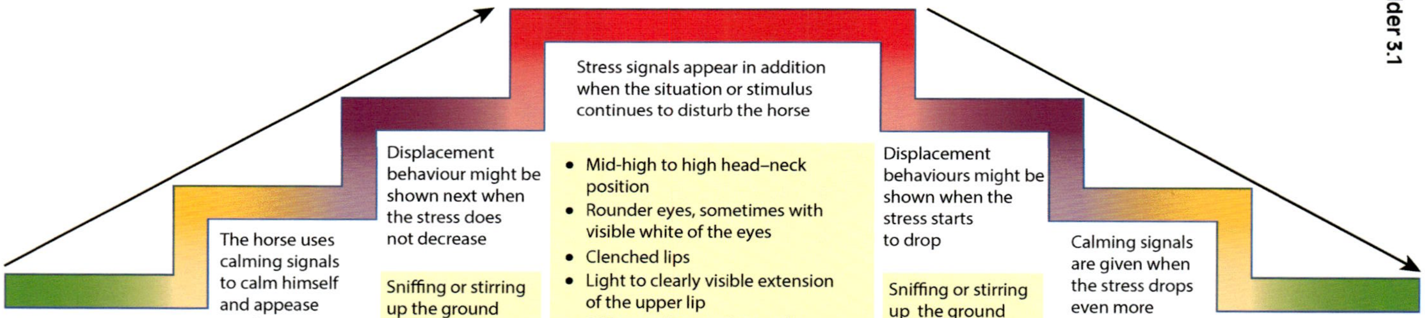

Stress increases because the situation changes due to a person, animal, sound or other stimulus in the environment

The horse uses calming signals to calm himself and appease another stimulus in the environment

Blinking; looking away; half closing the eyes; chewing; tongue out chewing; yawning; jaw stretch; head turn; neck turn; neck shake; body shake; see-saw lowering; sustained lowering; curving; splitting; showing the hindquarters; showing the flanks; eating; immobility and slowing down

Displacement behaviour might be shown next when the stress does not decrease

Sniffing or stirring up the ground without eating; rubbing the head/neck along own leg; rubbing the head/neck on objects; self-biting; licking objects; pawing; rolling; head swing

Stress signals appear in addition when the situation or stimulus continues to disturb the horse

- Mid-high to high head–neck position
- Rounder eyes, sometimes with visible white of the eyes
- Clenched lips
- Light to clearly visible extension of the upper lip
- Different shapes of upper lip and nose
- More visible 'curb' chin
- Rounder nostrils
- Actively moving ears
- Carried or clenched tail
- More frequent defecation and urination
- Pacing when obstructed
- Rushing: reduced eating or drinking, or unable to eat or drink
- Hasty movements
- Head swing
- More frequent startle reactions

Displacement behaviours might be shown when the stress starts to drop

Sniffing or stirring up the ground without eating; rubbing the head/neck along own leg; rubbing the head/neck on objects; self-biting; licking objects; pawing; rolling; head swing

Calming signals are given when the stress drops even more

Blinking; looking away; half closing the eyes; chewing; tongue out chewing; yawning; jaw stretch; head turn; neck turn; neck shake; body shake; see-saw lowering; sustained lowering; curving; splitting; showing the hindquarters; showing the flanks; eating; immobility and slowing down

Stress decreases because the calming signals are working, and/or the stimulus that is causing the stress disappears, and/or a person or animal changes his behaviour, and/or the horse recognises the situation and is able to handle it

3.3 BODY POSTURE AND FACIAL FEATURES

When a horse's tension is rising, you can tell this is the case from a number of important features:

- The head–neck position moves between mid-high and high (**Fig. 3.1**).
- The horse's muscles become increasingly tense.
- Facial features such as the nose and eyes reflect the tension. The higher the tension, the rounder the nose and eyes become simultaneously.
- The tail is carried in a light to high position or is clenched.
- In case of higher tension, the mouth and nose assume different shapes.

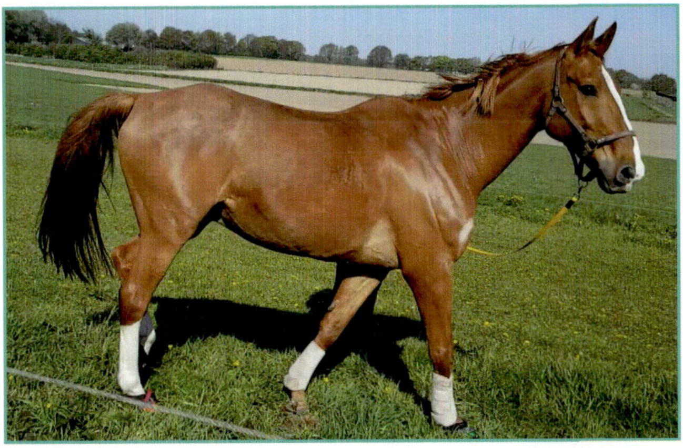

Fig. 3.1 This horse is showing a head–neck position between mid-high and high as he experiences tension. Other tension features are also shown.

ROUNDER EYES REFLECT TENSION

The horse's eyes are rounder and sometimes you can see some of the whites of the eyes. This becomes visible because the horse opens his eyes wider in order to see better (note that in horses whose eyes always show an edge of white around the iris, you will see more white because the eye is opened further). The eyes of the same horse are shown (**Figs 3.2–3.4**).

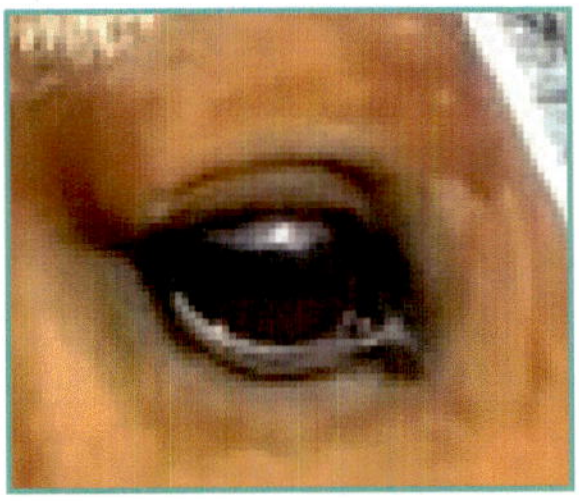

Fig. 3.2 Relaxed almond-shaped eye.

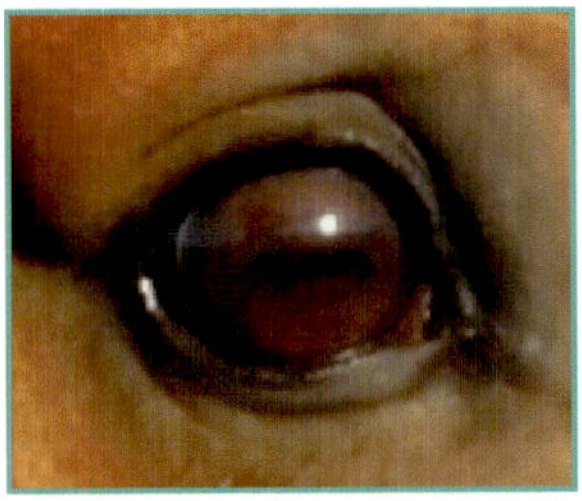

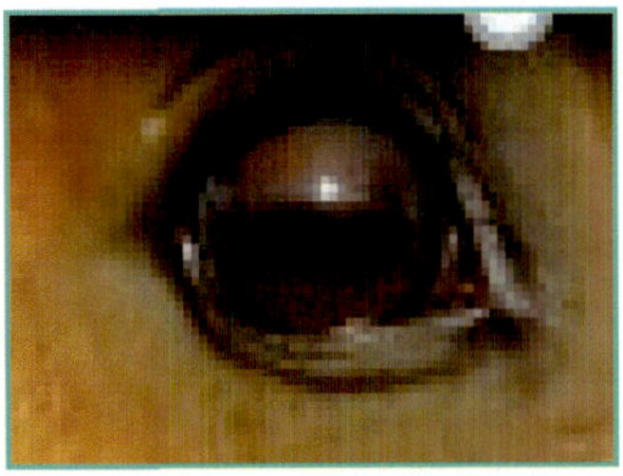

Figs 3.3, 3.4 Round tense eye.

ROUNDER NOSTRILS REFLECT TENSION

The horse has rounder nostrils. These may be nostrils that contract from round to long and back, or nostrils that stay round. The nose of the same horse photographed on two different occasions is shown (**Figs 3.5, 3.6**).

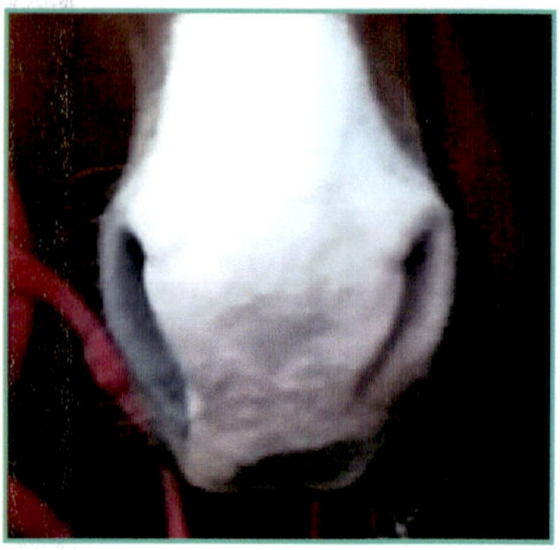

Fig. 3.5 Relaxed long nostrils.

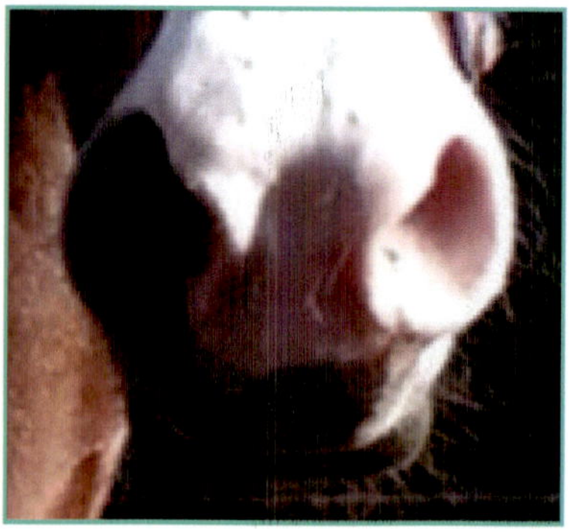

Fig. 3.6 Tense round nostrils.

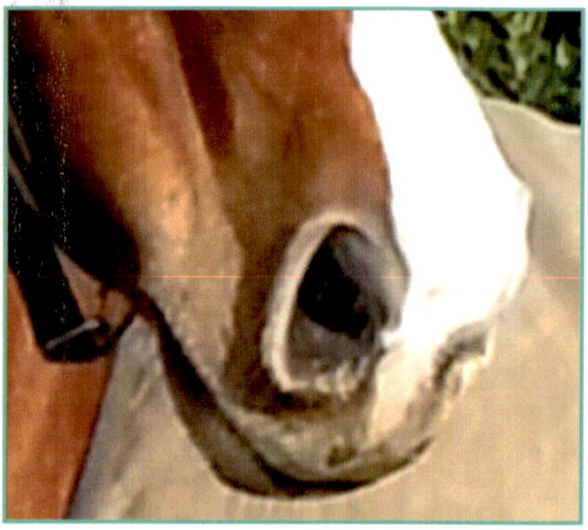

Fig. 3.7 Sagging nostril.

NOTE: A horse who has been running fast or working hard, or has been doing scent work, can also have round nostrils, which indicates that the horse needs a greater intake of air or oxygen. If this is the case, the horse shows no other signs of tension. He will also not have shown any calming signals or displacement behaviour. If a horse has been running hard for a long time with round nostrils, the nostrils can start to sag a little with the exertion (**Fig. 3.7**).

TAIL POSTURE

When tension is rising the tail dock will range between a lightly carried tail and a highly carried tail (**Figs 3.8–3.13**).

NOTE: You may also see a lightly carried tail when the horse is relaxed but needs to balance his body when riding or working. Additionally, you may see a lightly carried tail on a relaxed horse when the tail needs to be put to work, for example, to swipe away flies.

The tail also indicates tension when it is tightly clenched to the hindquarters (**Figs 3.14, 3.15**).

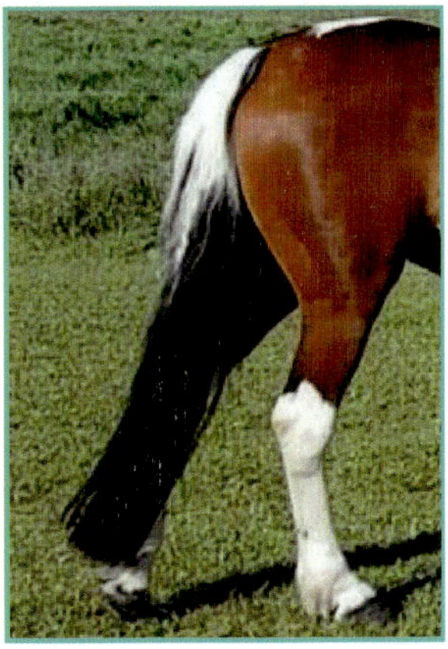

Fig. 3.8 Relaxed tail.

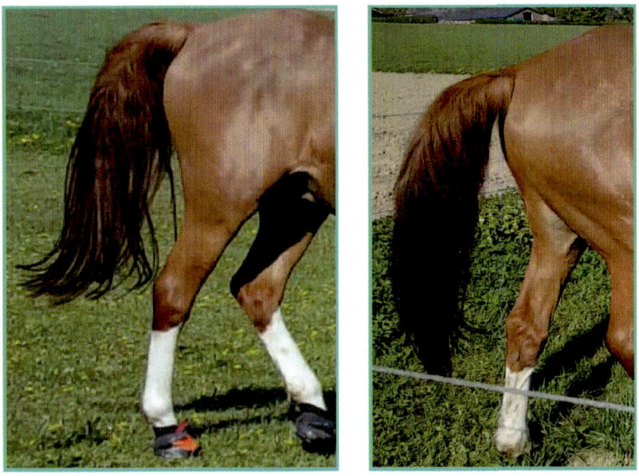

Figs 3.9, 3.10 Lightly carried tail.

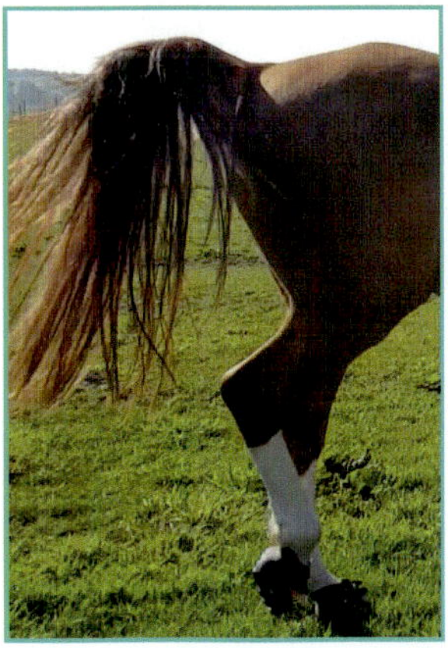

Fig. 3.11 Moderately carried tail.

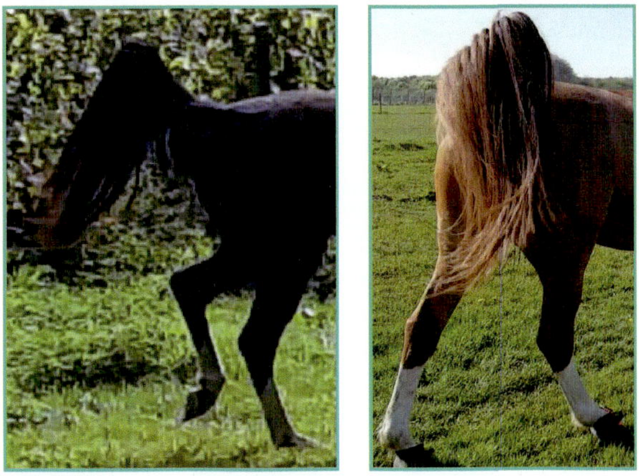

Figs 3.12, 3.13 Highly carried tail.

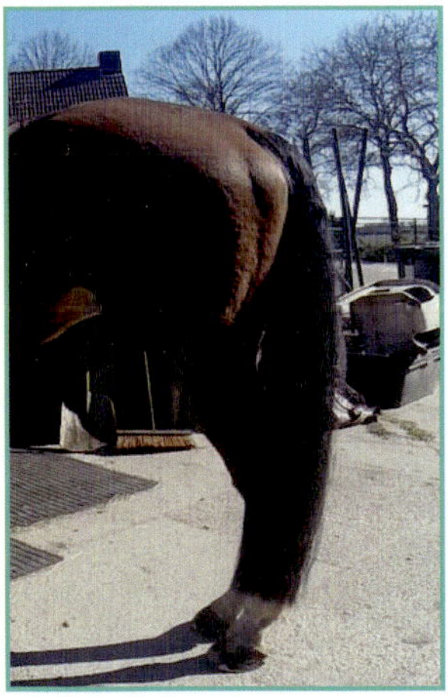

Fig. 3.14 A more relaxed tail.

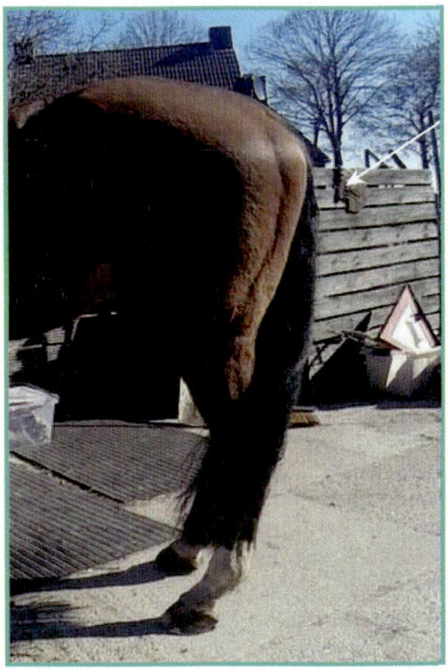

Fig. 3.15 A clenched tail.

3.4 CLENCHED LIPS AND DIFFERENTLY SHAPED LIPS AND NOSE

The mouth is a good measure of a horse's tension. A relaxed mouth has a relaxed lower lip (**Fig. 3.16**). The corner of the lower lip may protrude slightly in front of the upper lip or the rim of the lower lip may be visible. The lower lip may also be slightly longer than the upper lip (but note that this is also often a physical feature of older horses).

When a horse is becoming slightly tense, you will see him tighten his lips. One lip is no longer more extended than the other, but they connect seamlessly and may even be clenched (**Fig. 3.17**).

If the tension then rises even further, you will see that the upper lip can assume different shapes. It may, for example, become longer and protrude in front of the lower lip or it may be extended like a flute, or, contrarily, it may be drawn tightly against the teeth. Of course, the nose will move in different ways with these movements of the upper lip.

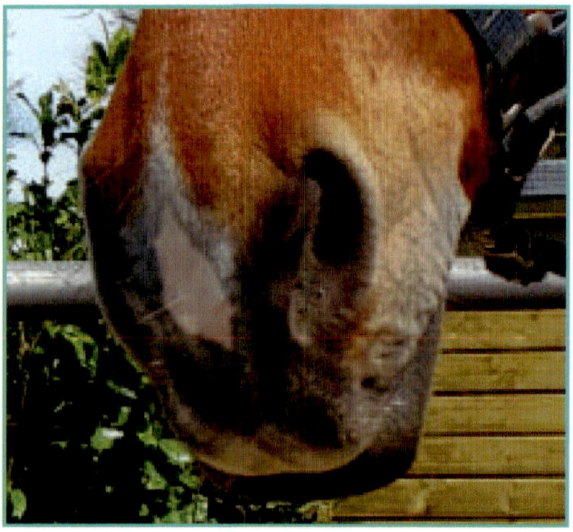

Fig. 3.16 A relaxed mouth.

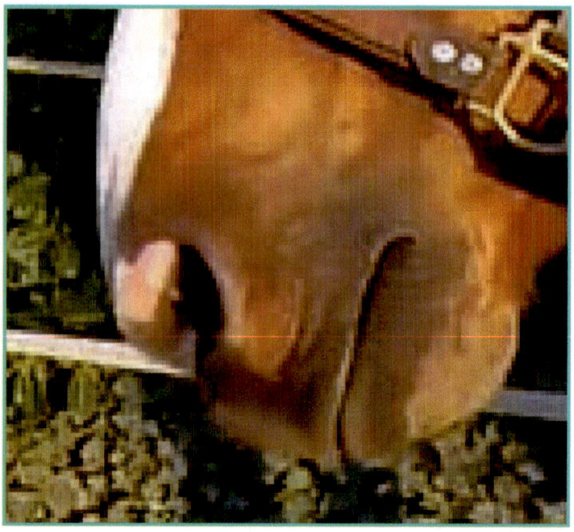

Fig. 3.17 A tense mouth with clenched lips.

Different shapes of the lips and nose also reflect tension (**Figs 3.18–3.21**).

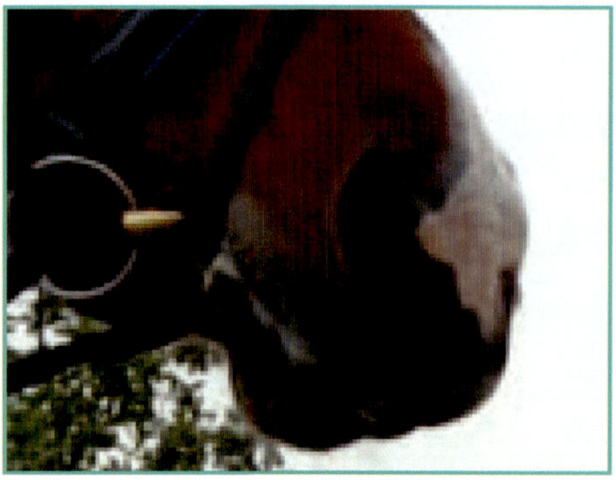

Fig. 3.18 Lengthened upper lip.

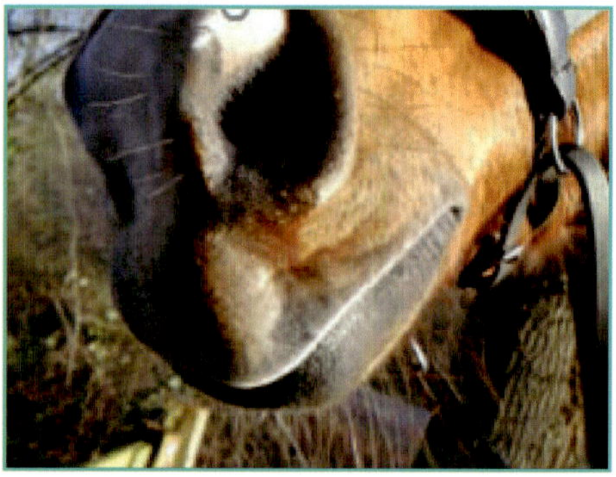

Fig. 3.19 Pointed nose.

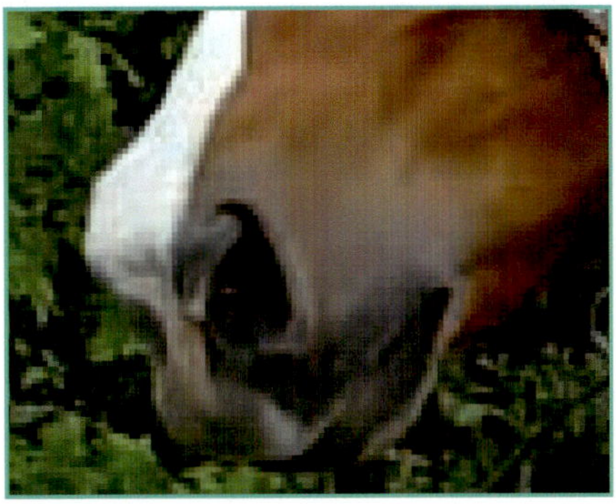
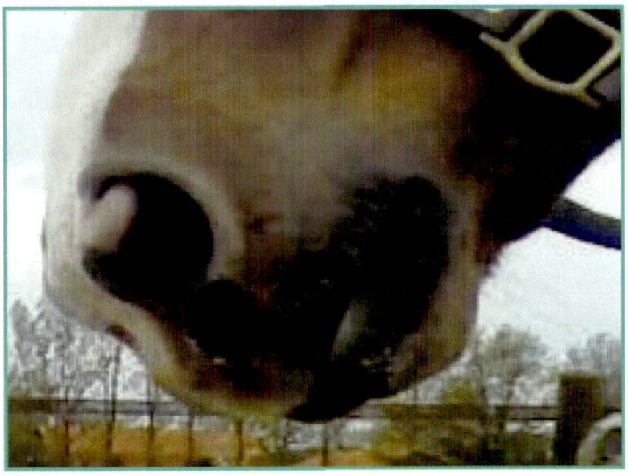

Figs 3.20, 3.21 Concave nose.

A TENSE NOSE AND MOUTH: A PHYSICAL EXERTION

A tense nose and mouth and a protruding upper lip may also be seen before a horse uses them as a tool (**Figs 3.22, 3.23**), for example, when a horse intends to eat something such as a leaf off a tree or grass off the ground, or if he intends to pick something up, or give a small push or bite threat (see section 3.11).

You may also see a tense mouth and protruding upper lip when a horse intends to groom himself or another horse or when you are grooming your horse on his favourite spots.

The use of the mouth is sometimes indicated by wrinkles appearing around the nose. This may be in between the nostrils and on the side of his mouth above the upper lip. When a horses uses his mouth as a tool he might be relaxed or tense.

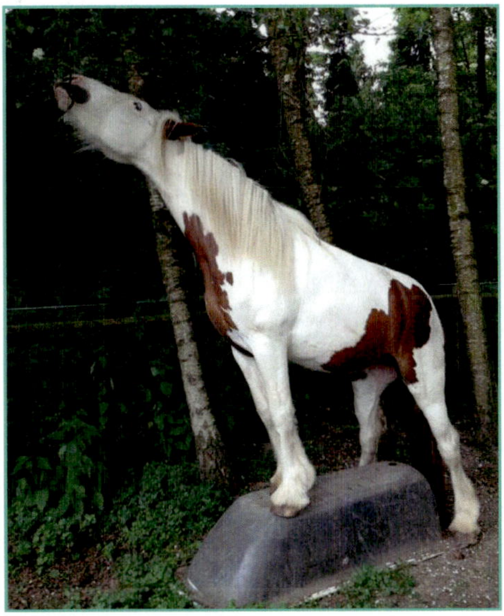
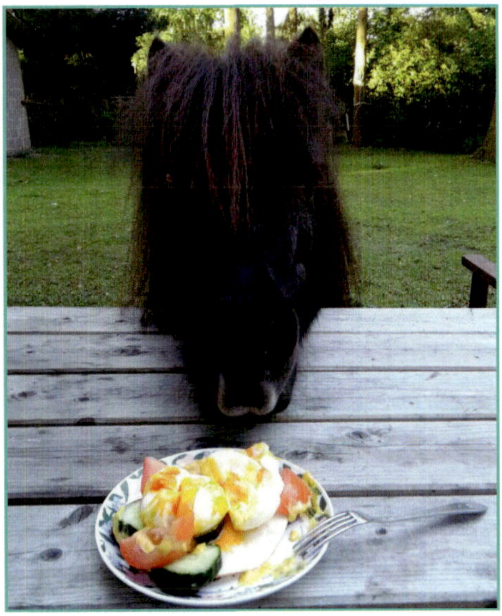

Figs 3.22, 3.23 Examples of extended upper lips being used as a tool.

Other tension features that can sometimes be seen include: the molars may be clenched, producing a line or a thickening in the area that extends beyond the seam of the mouth; the corners of the mouth may be pulled up, making the seam of the mouth look longer; the veins in the face may also be more visible; and the curb groove may no longer seem to blend into the chin in a straight line but assume a more pronounced 'cup-like' shape (**Figs 3.24, 3.25**).

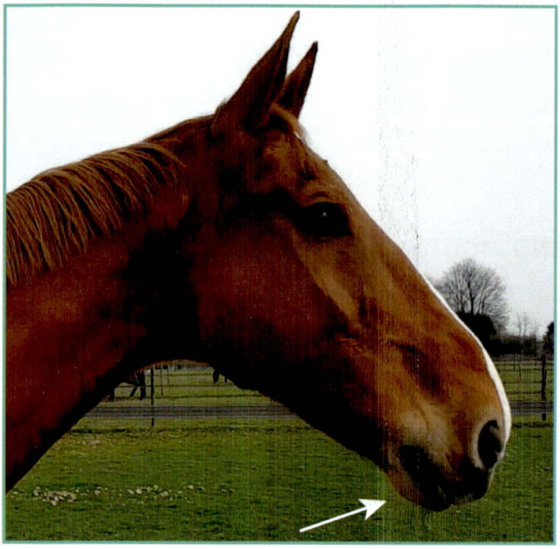

Fig. 3.24 Relaxed chin.

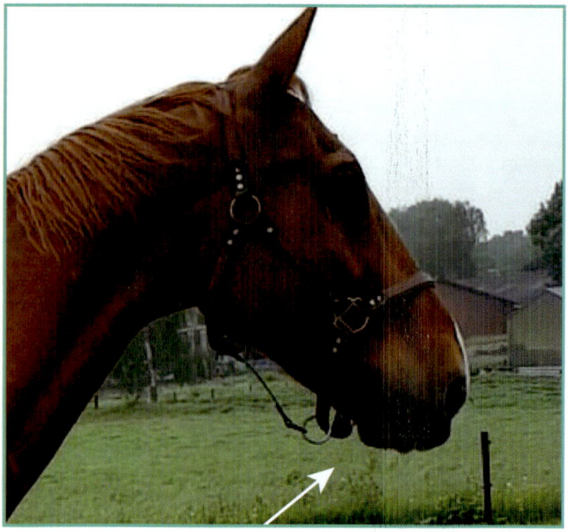

Fig. 3.25 A more tense 'cup'-shaped chin.

NOTE: In horses who naturally have a cup-shaped chin when they are relaxed, you will see that it is tensed when the horse feels tension. When this happens, the softer cup-shaped chin is drawn into a more pointed shape.

When you are with your horse and you notice that one of his features is tense – his nostrils, eyes, or tail, for example – you should look at his other features to determine if they are also shaped in a way that indicates tension. The more elements you see that reflect tension simultaneously, the higher the tension level of your horse. When this happens, try to figure out which stimulus or stimuli are causing it. **Figure 3.26** lists the tension features of the eyes, nose, mouth, and tail of the horse, because these are easily visible.

State	Head position	Nose, eyes, mouth	Tail
Relaxed	All head–neck positions are possible	Nostrils long, eyes almond-shaped and mouth relaxed. A rim or corner of the lower lip may be visible	Tail is relaxed, hangs loosely
Light tension	All head–neck positions are possible	Nose and/or eyes round/tense, mouth relaxed and loosely closed	Tail is relaxed or carried lightly
Medium tension	Mid-high to high head–neck positions	Nose and/or eyes round/tense, mouth tense	Tail is carried lightly to moderate
High tension	High head–neck position	Nose and eyes round/tense, mouth clenched, and possibly a differently shaped upper lip, nose or a cup-shaped chin	Tail is carried lightly to high

Fig. 3.26 Tension features of the nose, eyes, mouth, and tail in different states of tension.

Have a look at these faces of the same horse, photographed in three different situations (**Figs 3.27–3.29**).

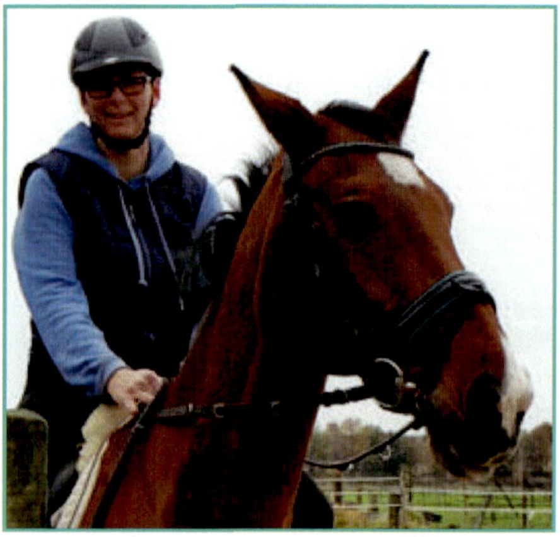

Fig. 3.27 Gertie is riding Orion. She stops to have this photo taken. Orion is standing in the arena. His nostrils are round. His eyes are almond-shaped and relaxed. His mouth is relaxed; his lips are not clenched. Orion is showing a state of light tension. One facial feature is tense: the round nostrils. This could also be due to physical exertion.

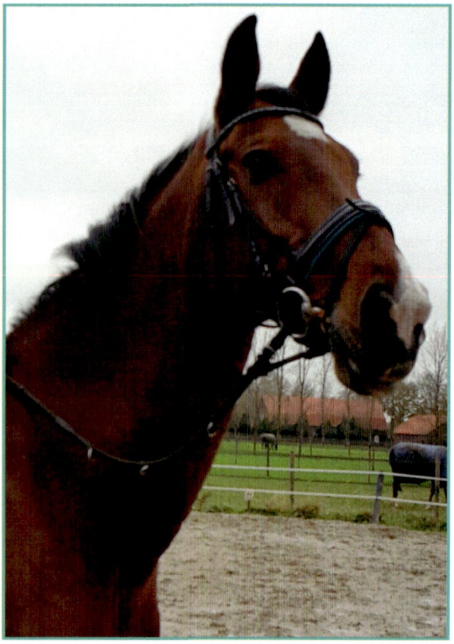

Fig. 3.28 Orion is being photographed in the arena on a different day. He looks at me as I walk over bushes to approach and take the photo. His eyes and nostrils are round. His lips are not clenched. Orion is showing a state of medium tension. Two features out of three, the eyes and the nose, are tense, the mouth is not.

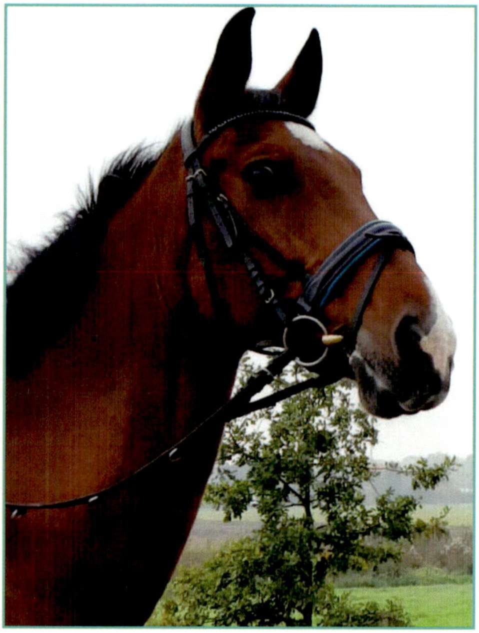

Fig. 3.29 Orion is being photographed while riding in the country. He is standing still and hears something. He has the highest head–neck position. His nostrils are round and stay round as he breathes. His upper lip slides over his lower lip. His eye is round. The white of the eye is showing. In this photo Orion is showing a state of high tension Three out of three features (eyes, nose, and mouth) are tense. In addition, the upper lip is extended.

Other horses have now been photographed in different situations (**Figs 3.30–3.37**).

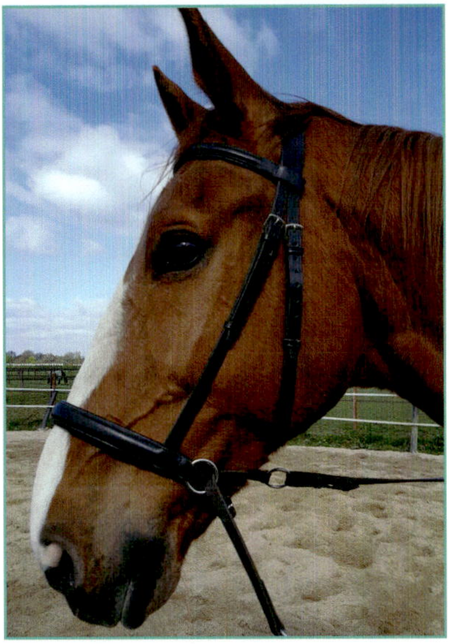

Fig. 3.30 Vosje and I are back from a ride in the country. Vosje's nostrils are round from exertion. His eyes are almond-shaped and relaxed. His mouth is also relaxed. (Light tension.)

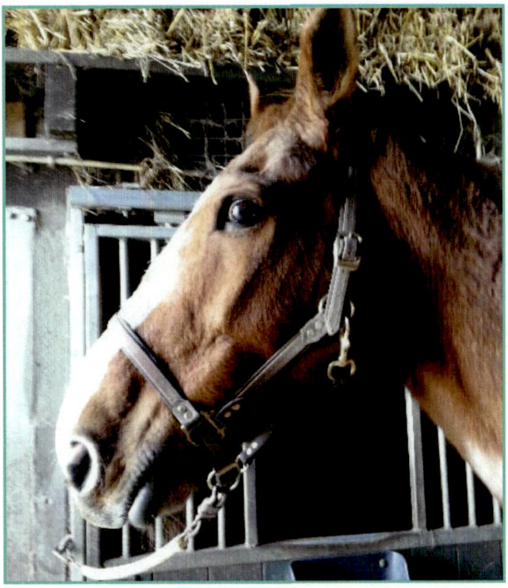

Fig. 3.31 Vosje is tied up in the grooming area. He hears the sound of a Bobcat coming from his left. His ear turns towards the sound. He looks sideways, in the direction of the sound. His eye is round and tense and opened more than usual. You can even see a sliver of white in his eye. His nostrils are also round. His upper lip is extended and slides over the lower lip slightly. In the area that extends beyond the seam of the mouth, you can see a thickening take shape because Vosje is clenching his jaws. (High tension.)

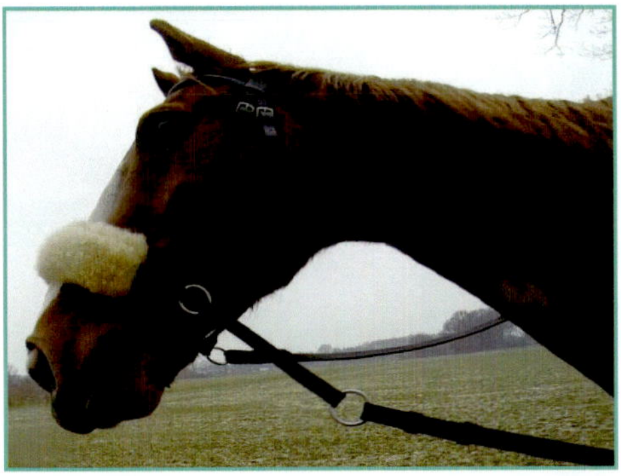

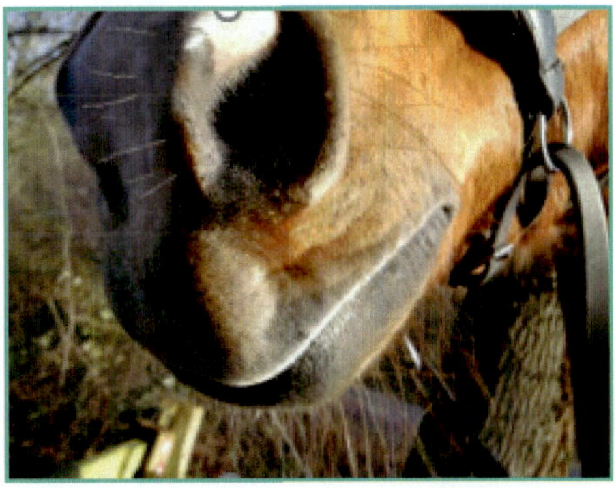

Figs 3.32, 3.33 I am hand walking Vosje outside. We pass a bus. There is high tension. Vosje's eyes are round, his nostrils are dilated, and his upper lip is extended. Because of the dilated nostrils and extended upper lip, an extra dip appears just below the nostrils, over the upper lip (Fig. 3.33).

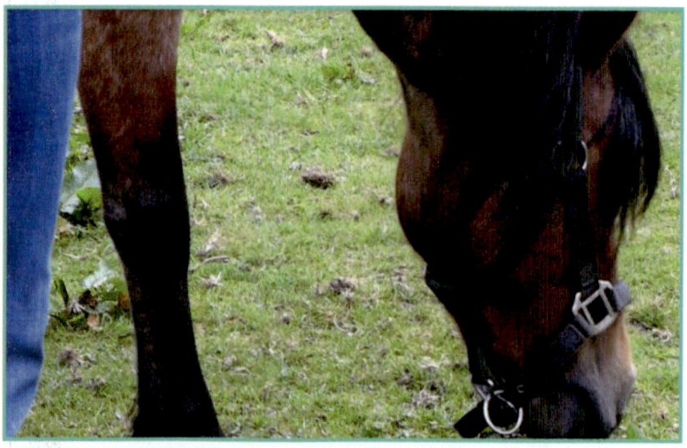

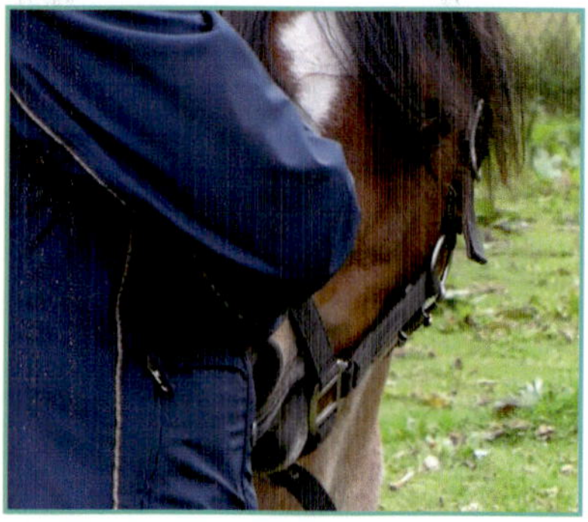

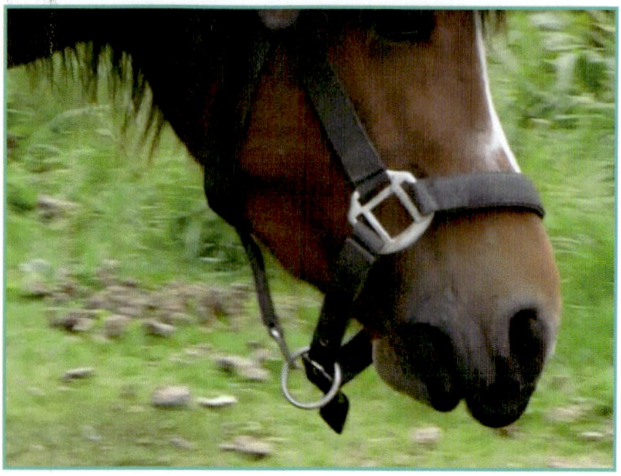

Fig. 3.34–3.36 ***Top left:*** I walk over to Indy and stop by her shoulder. Just a part of my leg is shown. ***Top right:*** Indy turns towards me to figure out what she will do next. ***Left:*** Indy walks away, showing a lot of tension in her upper lip. Both her eyes and nostrils are round. The upper lip may also be extended because she starts to resume her grazing after a few seconds, and an extended upper lip is an indication of this. It can also be a combination of both.

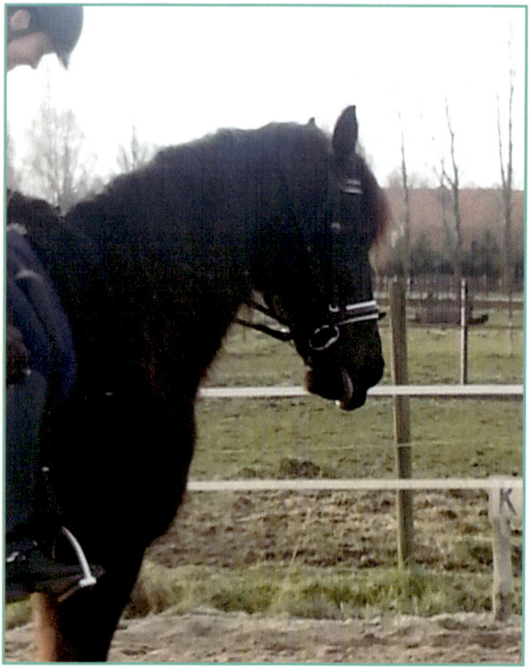

Fig. 3.37 While being ridden, horses may extend their upper lip when they are doing something or about to do something that is physically or cognitively difficult.

3.5 MORE FREQUENT DEFECATION AND URINATION

The function of defecation is indisputable. It is the anal excretion of indigestible foods, liquids, and other substances such as bacteria and dead body cells. Dung that is excreted when a horse is not tense is the size of a molehill. Dung consists of smaller parts that lump together.

A horse who is experiencing rising tension will, at moments when the tension rises, start to defecate more often. Because the cortisol level is raised and, with it, the hormone corticotropin, colon motility increases through colonic contractions, which leads to an increased stool output and transit speed.[10]

Tension will also cause a horse to urinate more frequently.[11] This might be something you will see more often in horses who are not being ridden and who can urinate more freely, without the added restrictions of the riding gear or possible negative associations taught to them by riders who do not want their horses to urinate or defecate while riding or hand walking.

Defecation and urination due to tension occur when the horse is actually feeling that tension (**Figs 3.38–3.44**). His head–neck position is mid-high to high, his face shows signs of tension, and he carries his tail lightly. If there is increasing tension, you will first see the horse show calming signals and displacement behaviour before he starts to defecate. If there is a sudden shock or high tension, the horse may skip the calming signals and displacement activities and go straight to defecation. This is because there is no build-up of tension, but the tension suddenly appears, without any warning.

A horse who defecates due to tension often wants to convert tension into movement, often a flight motion. If the handler or rider prevents this, you will see the horse defecate at a slow trot or while moving back and forth when tied up. A horse who defecates due to tension does so differently to when he is relaxed. Sometimes the tension causes the horse to lift and hold his tail high for a few

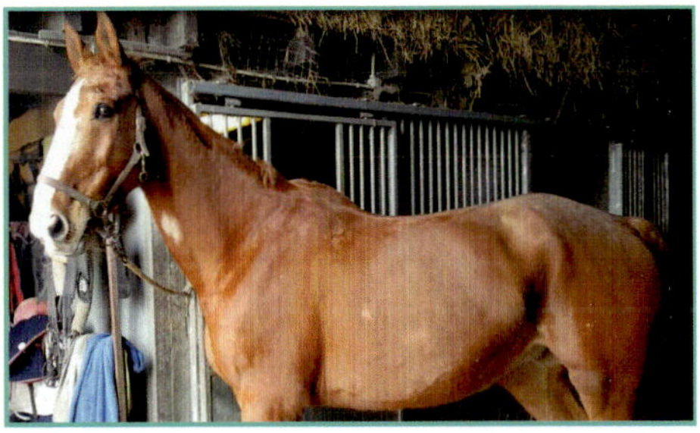

Fig. 3.38 Vosje is tied up. He hears an unfamiliar sound coming from outside. He feels tension, which is clearly visible on his face. He has round eyes and nostrils. His tail is also lightly raised. His ears are pointed in the direction of his attention. He blinks a few times as a calming signal (not visible in the photo).

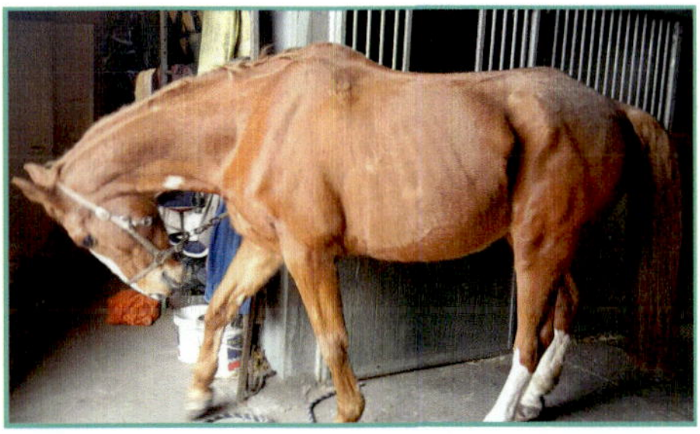

Fig. 3.39 Vosje paws. This is displacement behaviour, which I believe may also indicate that he wants to leave the situation and walk away in the direction of his scraping and stance.

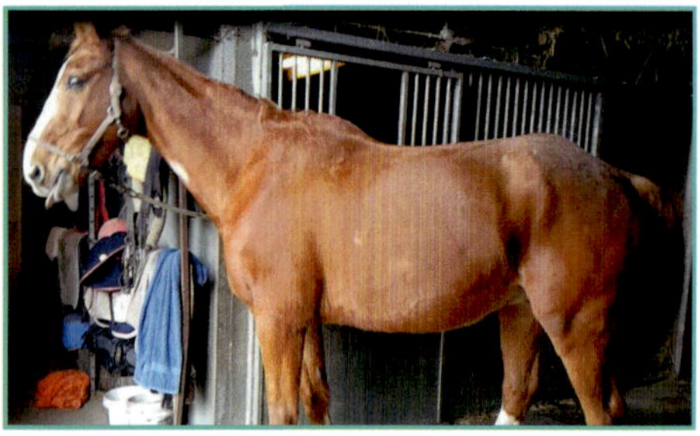

Fig. 3.40 As a calming signal, Vosje shows tongue out chewing.

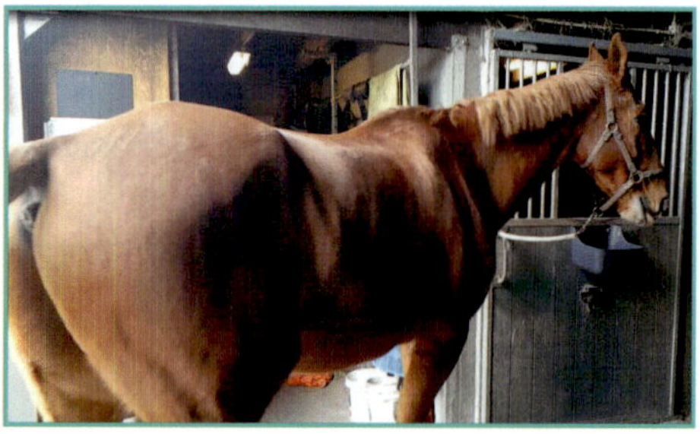

Fig. 3.41 Vosje turns on the rope. He turns his hindquarters towards the noise and then turns back to his original position again right away. The showing of the hindquarters may in this case be a sign of anxiety, a calming signal, or a combination of both. He chews as a calming signal. The tail is lightly carried.

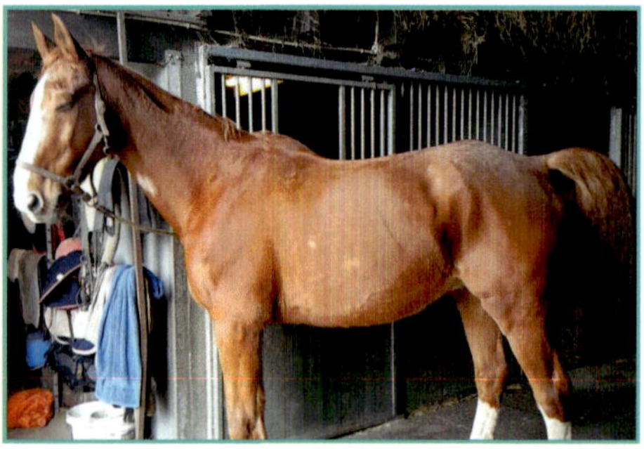

Fig. 3.42 Vosje blinks.

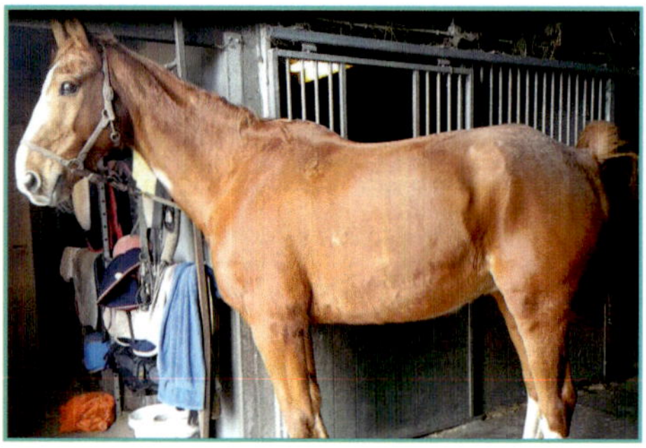

Fig. 3.43 Vosje defecates due to tension.

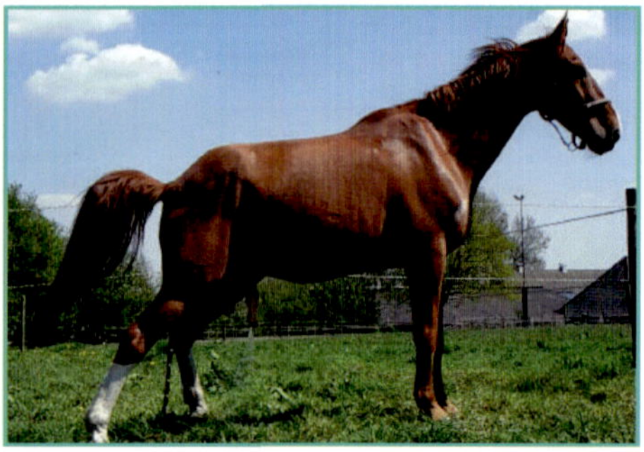

Fig. 3.44 Vosje is at pasture in a new location. He urinates six times in two hours. These are short, hurried urinations. Sometimes the penis has not even come out of its sheath before he urinates.

seconds before possibly defecating. Sometimes the anus only excretes a little fluid; sometimes it immediately excretes dung. The amount of dung is often smaller than when the horse is relaxed. It may be only one small part, or the dung may be less formed and less neatly divided into smaller clumps. The dung may also look like a formless goo. When the horse is moving back and forth, the dung is spread out in small quantities.

3.6 RUSHING: EATING, DRINKING, AND MOVING

It is a good idea to examine how your horse eats and drinks when he is relaxed. This way, you will have comparison material for when your horse starts to build up tension, because the higher the tension, the more hurriedly your horse will do these things.

He will move back and forth more as he eats and drinks. He will regularly stop eating, raise his head to the high position to listen to sounds, look around, or call out. Sometimes he will let food drop out of his mouth. He uses faster chewing motions. As mentioned in section 2.20, the higher the tension, the higher the bite frequency. Sometimes there is also a change in biting technique. If the tension becomes too great, he will stop eating and drinking altogether and no longer accept food and water that is offered.

Ted is a 6-month-old Tinker. He has just arrived at a new stable. In the first days, he has a stall with an open top. He can see two horses and they can approach him. Ted is restless. Both his ears are pointed forward. He is making circles in his stall, stopping several times to listen, his head raised to the highest position and his face showing signs of high tension. He sometimes calls out to the other horses. After circling and doing 'listening stops' for half an hour, he stands still. His ears are still hard at work though. They rotate and keep going from the front to the side to the back, over and over again. As Ted settles down and starts to understand his surroundings, his ear movements also calm down.

In this scenario it is first the body movements that are fast, then the ear movements show a fast pattern, and finally the emotional rest translates into physical rest.

You also see rushed movements when a horse slow jogs when being ridden or hand walked. In this situation the restrictions imposed by the rider or handler cause the slow jogging. Had the horse been loose, he would have acted on his own impulses and the gait that went with them. It is true in this case as well: an emotionally restless horse immediately incorporates this into his movements.

PACING

Pacing is a regular feature of the lives of domesticated horses. I see that many horse lovers consider this to be fairly normal and acceptable behaviour on the part of the horse. A horse paces when a barrier separates him from the place, animal, or person he wants to get to. Because the horse cannot pass the barrier but wants to go to the place of his choice, you will see him start to walk, trot, or canter (depending on his internal motivation and level of tension) along the barrier. He holds his head mid-high to high as he does this, and he keeps looking at the place, animal, or object he wants to get to. Both his ears are pointed that way too, regardless of whether he is moving clockwise or counter-clockwise.

The level of tension in a horse who is pacing may be different. This is directly expressed in his behaviour. If the horse walks past the fence a couple of times, shows a few calming signals, then walks off to graze, he has been feeling tension from which he could recover by himself.

However, the horse's internal motivation to go somewhere may also be strong, appealing directly to his underlying needs and fears. A horse may pace because he cannot be alone and wants to stay with other horses. The horse may be in pain, hungry, or cold, and that is why he wants to go to the stable. He may have become fearful and wants to return to the stable, where it is safe. Perhaps other horses were brought back to the stable first, leaving him the last one out there. All of these situations incur tension. I think, therefore, that pacing is not something that should be ignored. You should gauge if the horse is able to recover on his own after light tension or if he is dealing with high tension that he cannot overcome on his own. If that is the case, the handler should help, identify the cause, and make a practice plan.

3.7 EXAMPLE OF A BEHAVIOUR SEQUENCE

Tension can also manifest very subtly. The three photos below were taken at 1-second intervals (**Figs 3.45–3.47**).

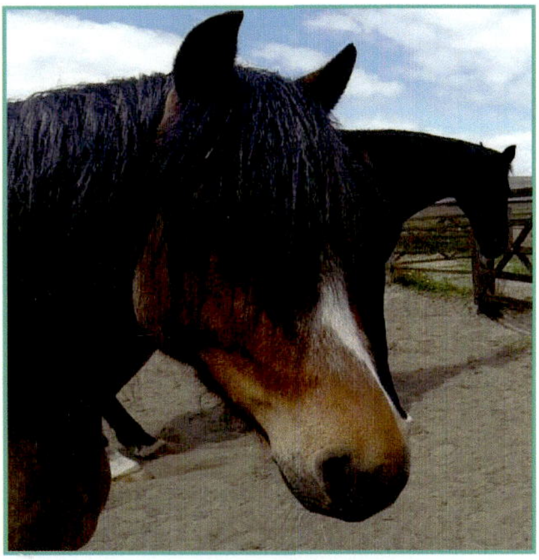

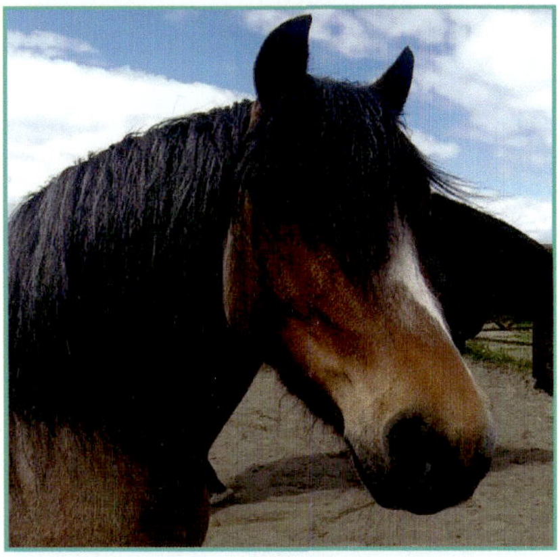

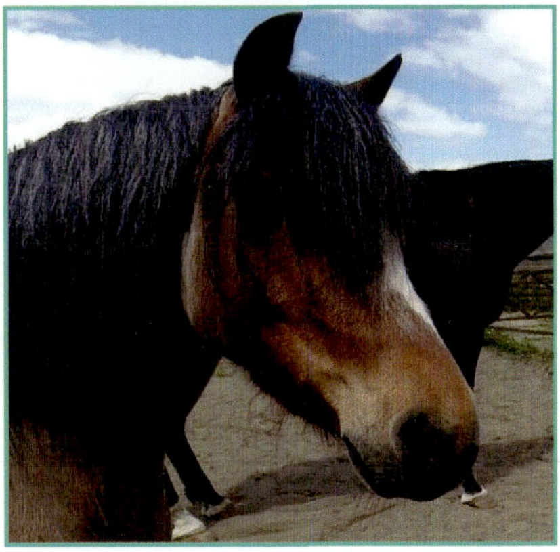

Figs 3.45–3.47 ***Top:*** I am standing still. Indy is looking at me. ***Middle:*** I take a step towards Indy. On the first step, she lifts her head higher. Her eyes become rounder, even showing a bit of white. Her nostrils also become rounder. The upper lip seems to protrude in front of the lower lip. ***Bottom:*** I am standing still. Indy recovers. This is discernible by her long nostrils and almond-shaped eyes. Her head–neck position is still high though.

3.8 TENSION LEADS TO CREATION OF DISTANCE

When the stimulus that is creating tension in the horse stays the same or becomes stronger, it has a direct effect on the horse. His tension also will stay the same or become greater. When this is the case, two things can happen:

1 The horse takes action and moves away from the stimulus, increasing the distance between himself and the stimulus.
2 The horse takes action and moves towards the stimulus. He uses signals to get the stimulus to go away, to stop, or at least not to come any closer. Therefore, the horse, by his own actions, actively tries to maintain or increase the distance between himself and the stimulus. He does this mainly by threatening.

The signals a horse uses to increase the distance between himself and a stimulus, whether by walking away or by warning away the other, I have called 'distance increasing signals'. There are several reasons why a horse uses distance increasing signals:

1 The horse is in pain or expects pain, causing him to want to increase the distance from a stimulus such as a person, animal, or object. For example, a horse who suffers from back pain may show a distance increasing signal when you place the saddle on his back or are about to do so, or when you are about to tighten the girth.
2 The horse is not used to the stimulus, for example, a person. He is fearful and does not trust it. He uses a distance increasing signal to this person, animal, object, or sound.
3 The horse has what is to him a valuable possession such as food, water, or another horse. He wants to maintain or increase the distance between others and both himself and this valuable object.

Pearl and Indy are at pasture. Indy is standing next to the water trough. Pearl looks at Indy. Pearl's ears are turned back, her nose is extended a little, and her eyes are open and unblinking. Pearl makes a forward motion with her nose, as if giving Indy a little push through the empty air. Indy responds right away and walks away. Pearl starts to drink.

Gertie and I are riding through the woods. Vosje and I are in front with Gertie and Orion behind us. We are walking. When Orion moves next to Vosje, Vosje glances his way. His ears are turned back and his eyes are focused on Orion without blinking. Orion responds by slowing down and walking behind Vosje again. After 500 metres, we turn right onto the path that leads home. The horses start to walk faster and Orion moves out from behind Vosje to walk beside him again. Vosje looks to the side, his ears turned back and his nose extended a little. Orion keeps walking. Vosje turns his head away and immediately turns it back to Orion, his teeth slightly exposed. He threatens to bite, but does not. Biting the air is as far as he goes. Orion slows down and starts to walk behind Vosje again.

The distance increasing signals reflect a horse's internal motivations and indicate the boundaries of what he is able to handle, allowing the other horse to see what is important to him and what he finds too difficult. This is not fixed. What the horse finds important will depend on his circumstances. For example, a single water trough in a bare paddock will be more important to him during the dry summer months than in the autumn, when there are also puddles of rainwater everywhere. What a horse is able to handle also depends on his physical and mental condition, the circumstances, and the training. These vary and may change over time.

When a horse gives distance increasing signals, he does not intend to wound the other horse or be wounded himself. He walks away or may threaten to kick or bite. If he does kick or bite, it is only a weakened form and goes no further than a kick or bite into air. He will not actually bite or kick another horse. Even when he moves away as a distance increasing signal, it is only a slow walk, trot, or canter, not a true flight as if his life depended on it.

If the distance increasing signals are not recognised or heeded and the tension rises, then the situation can escalate to actual fighting, including possible injuries and extreme flight responses (see section 3.18). In my research I have seen many distance increasing signals. If the distance increasing signals were exchanged between the horses themselves, they were also recognised and acted upon. Approaches were broken off, and the horse who walked away was left alone. This prevented escalation.

Before a horse gives distance increasing signals, he may show a moment of immobility.

I deliberately do not use the term 'threatening signals' for the distance increasing signals where a horse moves proactively towards the stressful stimulus. After all, the term 'threatening signals' seems to stimulate people to want to dominate the horse at that moment. 'What do you mean threatening? I will show him threatening.' This more quickly produces the inclination to punish. The term distance increasing signals stresses that the horse needs space, and should be given help in his training and socialisation instead of punishment.

WEAKENED DISTANCE INCREASING SIGNALS

While observing your horse, you may see him give very light or weakened forms of distance increasing signals. For example, a horse might keep another horse at bay by looking at him with his ears turned back for a second or two, instead of giving a stronger driving off signal. The horse does not need the stronger signal now. The other horse understands the weaker signal just fine. Possibly (but not necessarily) the first horse has given a much stronger signal in the past or matters have come to blows at some point. The weakened signal is then the result of a mutual 'understanding'.

You can also think of a horse who is being saddled and moves a few paces away from the rider. These paces then represent a weakened form of the distance increasing signal of fleeing. This too can be the remnant of flight behaviour that used to be stronger and is still present in a weakened form.

It may also be the case that the horse has learned that distance increasing signals such as fleeing or threatening do not work in certain situations, and that he still shows these signals in a weakened form, only to quickly abandon them again.

These weakened forms of distance increasing signals are smaller in movement and expression and can be given during or after calming signals or during or after displacement activities and stress signals.

DISTANCE INCREASING SIGNALS ARE SKIPPED

If a threat suddenly appears, the horse has no time to communicate or warn anyone else. He has to react immediately, and so that is what he does.

3.9 COMMUNICATION LADDER: DISTANCE INCREASING SIGNALS

Ladder 3.2

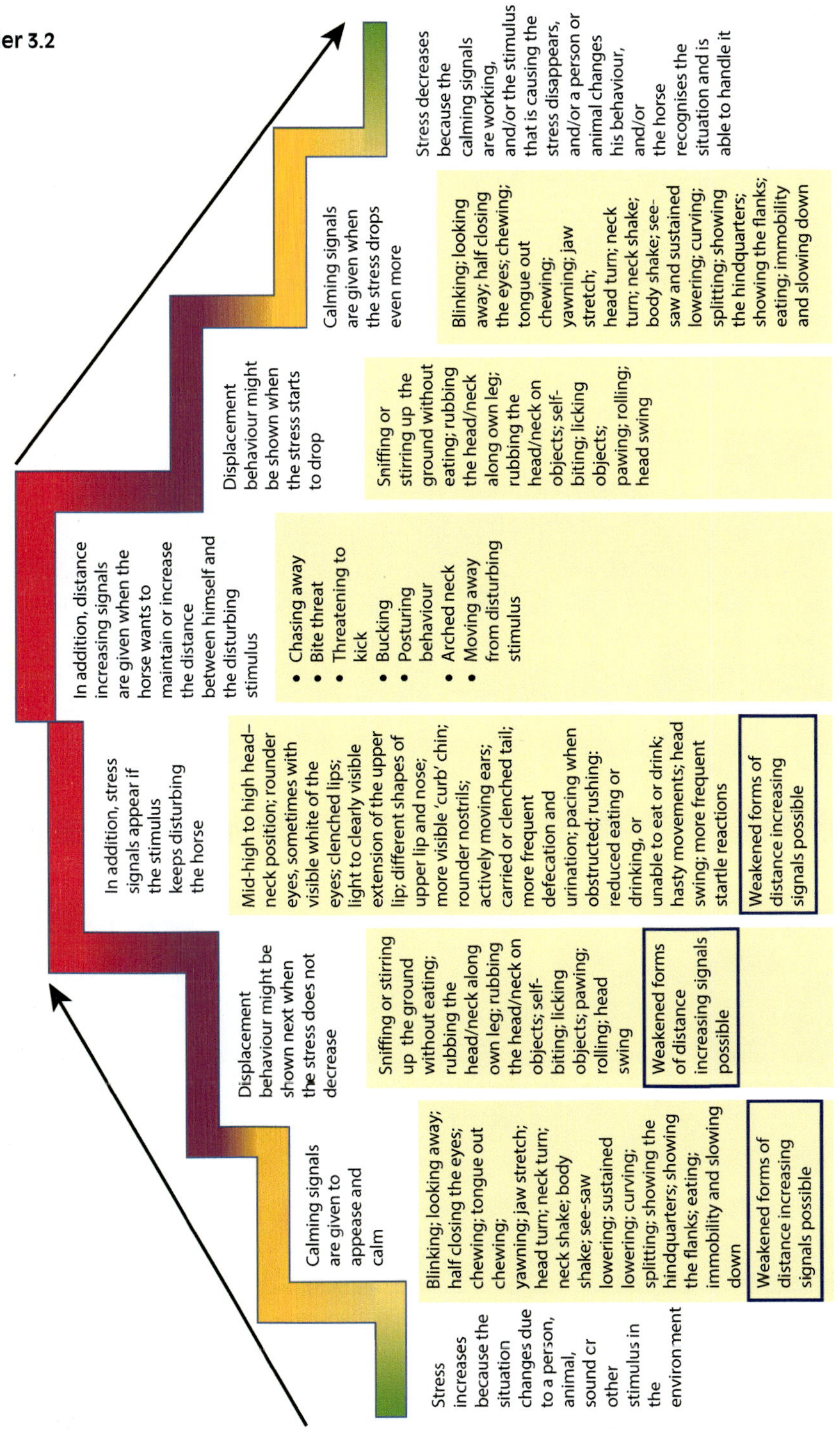

3.10 CHASING AWAY

Chasing away is the way a horse proactively increases the distance between himself and the other horse or between himself and the object he values (**Figs 3.48, 3.49**). The characteristic posture of a horse who is chasing away is:

- The head–neck position is between horizontal and high.
- The ears are pointed back or slightly pressed back.
- The eyes are kept open. They do not blink.
- The nose is pressed forwards a little. This can also be done with a movement in which the head is kept high and the horse almost nods and brings his nose back in, keeping the neck curled upwards slightly before pushing forwards again.
- A head swing can sometimes be seen as harbinger of a desire to drive others away.

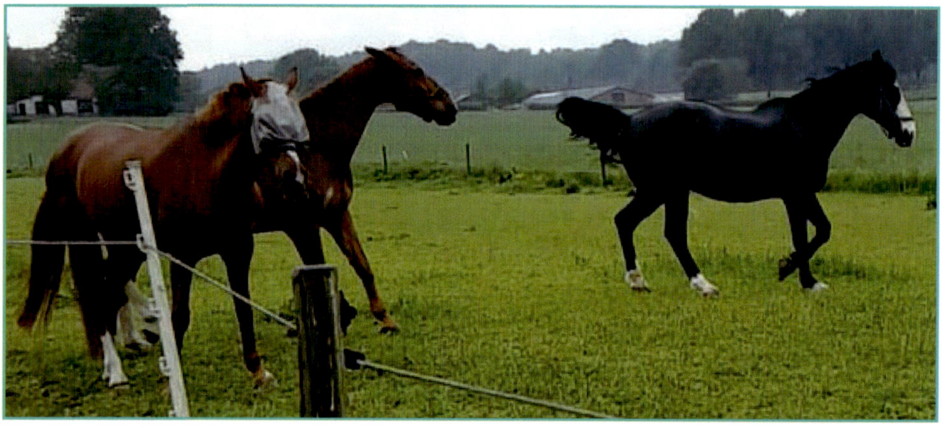

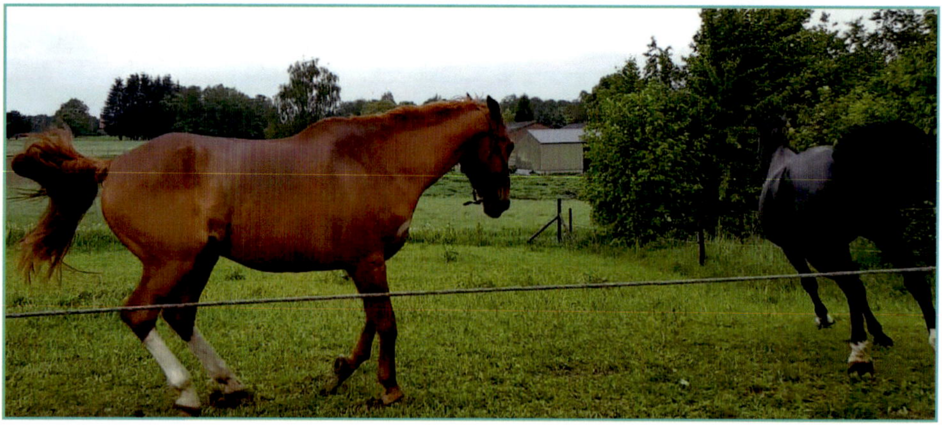

Figs 3.48, 3.49 ***Top:*** A distance increasing signal from the chestnut on the left (without a fly mask) towards the black horse. This is done from a walking gait and with a mild motivation. ***Bottom:*** In this photo the same horse is chasing the other horse away under higher tension.

3.11 BITE THREAT

When a horse uses a bite threat as a distance increasing signal, he is saying to the other horse, 'Stop what you are doing' or 'Stop, I need more space'. Threatening to bite as a distance increasing signal is characterised by the fact that the horse does not actually bite. It is a warning. The horse quickly turns his head sideways towards the one he is trying to warn, bears his teeth, opens his mouth slightly, and threatens to bite (possibly audibly clicking his teeth together) (**Figs 3.50, 3.51**). The ears can be in different positions for this. Both ears may be turned back or one ear may be pointed forward while the other is turned towards whoever the horse is communicating with. If the other horse does not heed the warning, how often the horse will keep giving the signal before he actually bites depends on the horse and the prevailing circumstances.

A bite threat and biting can also occur as a part of play, mutual grooming, or when examining objects. Horses may air bite or bite when they experience an unpleasant or painful stimuli, for instance if they experience a stab of pain such as when the girth is being tightened.

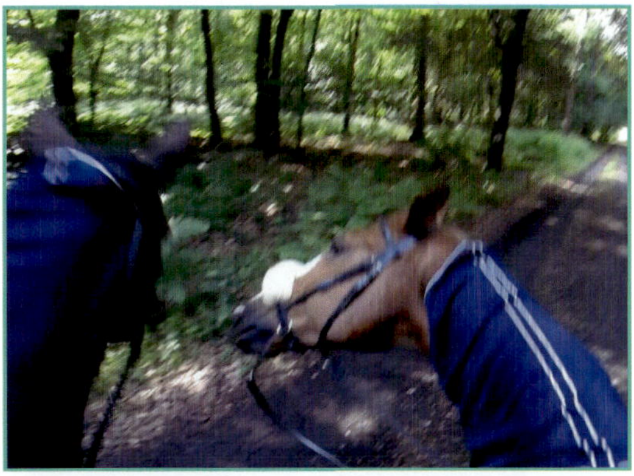

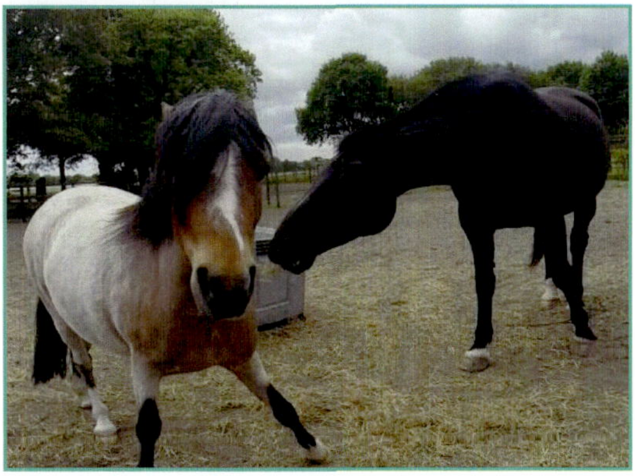

Figs 3.50, 3.51 ***Top:*** Vosje, the horse on the right, air bites in the direction of Orion, the horse on the left, when the latter increases his tempo and moves up beside Vosje. After Vosje's bite threat, Orion slows down and moves back behind Vosje again. ***Bottom:*** Indy, the pony on the left, wants to walk to her left but is stopped by Pearl. After Pearl air bites in Indy's direction, Indy turns right instead.

3.12 THREATENING TO KICK

Nothing is more effective at increasing the distance to other horses than threatening to kick with a hind leg or foreleg. Characteristic of kicking with a hind leg is the head being held in the highest position with the poll pressed into the neck a little. The nose is lifted slightly upwards and forwards. The facial features reflect medium to high tension (see **Fig. 3.26**). While threatening, the ears are turned sideways or back. In situations with the highest motivation and tension, the ears

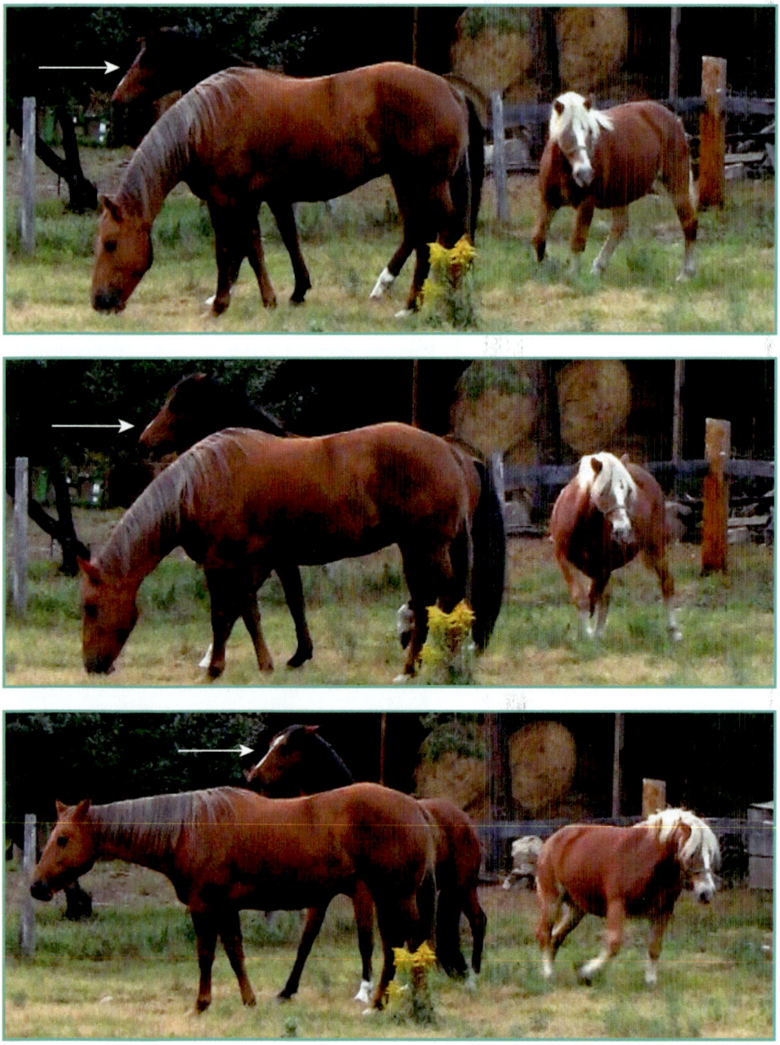

Figs 3.52–3.54 Dolly, the horse on the right in the photos, walks towards Benny (arrowed), the horse who is mostly hidden behind Flicka, the chestnut. Benny wants to stop Dolly's move. Dolly is coming too close. Benny gives a distance increasing signal. He threatens to kick. He also walks backwards a few paces as he does so. Dolly responds appropriately by increasing the distance between herself and Benny.

are pressed back. The horse turns his hindquarters to the one he wants to threaten, as if saying, 'Stop: no more'. Often the horse holds one hind leg slightly raised, threatening an actual kick. Walking backwards a few paces makes the threat even more effective (**Figs 3.52–3.54**). A horse can also look backwards without threatening (**Figs 3.55, 3.56**).

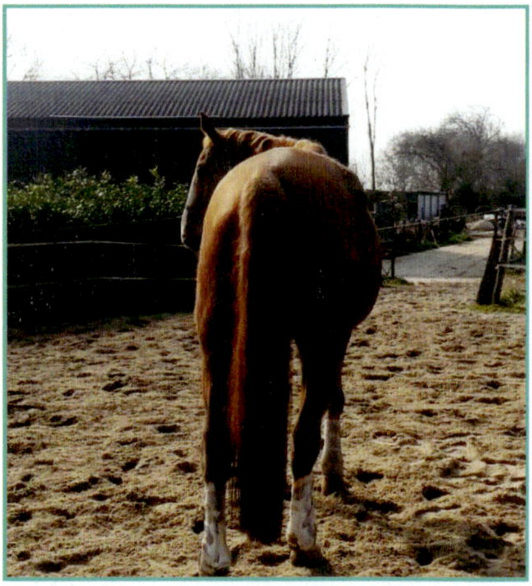

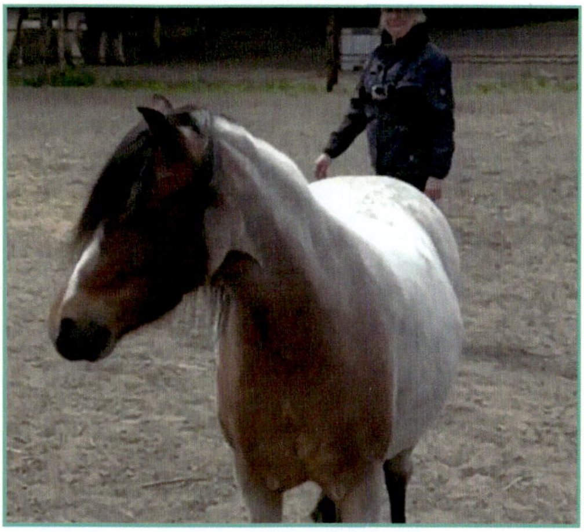

Figs 3.55, 3.56 These two photos are for comparison. Both horses look backwards, but these are not instances of distance increasing signals in the form of threatening to kick. The head–neck position is mid-high instead of high, the neck and back muscles are relaxed (the back looks long), the head is not tipped back, and with both horses one ear is turned back and the other forwards towards whoever they are trying to contact.

An arched neck is characteristically a warning of a kick with a foreleg (see section 3.14), during which the splenius capitis muscle remains tensed and both ears face forwards. If a foreleg kick follows, both ears turn back during the kick. The horse may also give a high-pitched scream. As a distance increasing signal, the foreleg kick is not a kick that actually connects. It serves as an intimidation move that does not actually touch the other party (**Figs 3.57–3.64**).

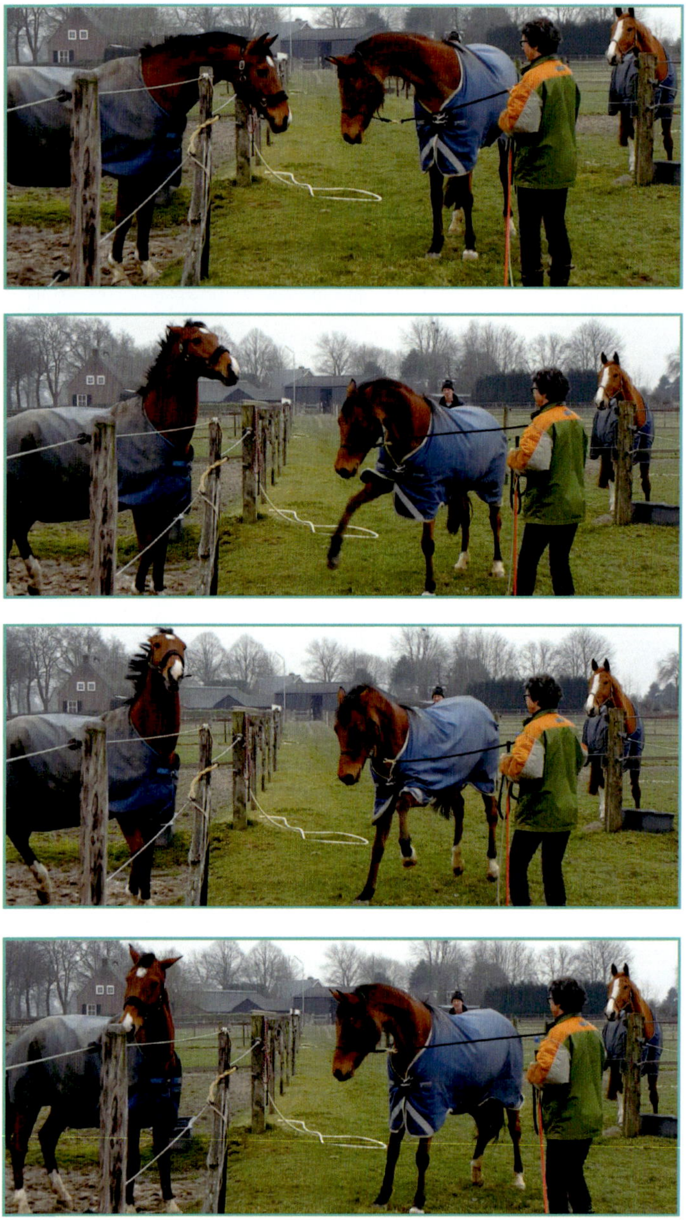

Figs 3.57–3.60 Marian is trying to see if the mare, Leah, on the right is in heat for breeding purposes. She is held in front of the gelding, Orion. ***Top***: You see Leah arching her neck. Both ears face forwards and her attention is focused on the gelding. ***Upper middle:*** Here you see Leah kicking with her foreleg. Both of her ears are turned back as she does this, and her upper lip is extended. Orion gives a flight response, both ears turned back. The seam of his mouth is long. ***Lower middle:*** This shows the mare kicking with her foreleg and doing small jumps into the air with her hind legs. Leah lands squarely. In the meantime, Orion does a neck turn. In the video footage you can then see both horses giving calming signals. ***Bottom:*** Leah chews and blinks. Orion does a neck turn.

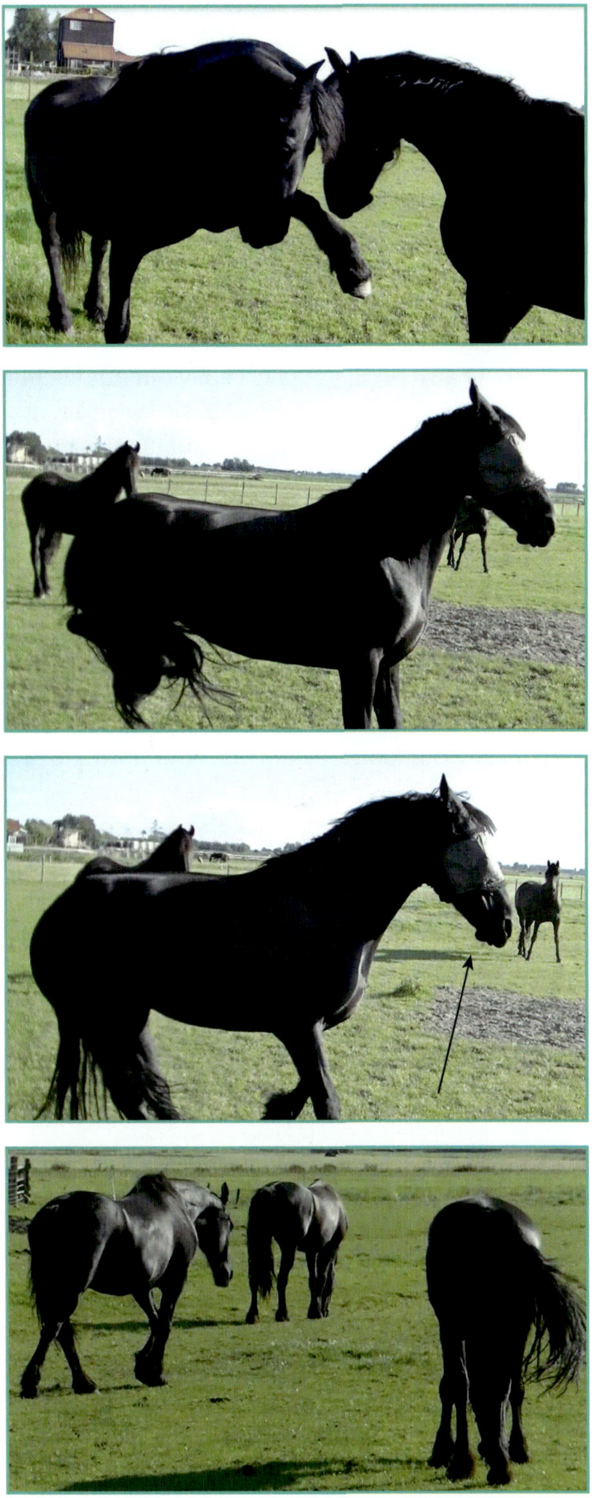

Figs 3.61–3.64 ***Top:*** The horse on the right is released into a paddock. He walks up to the horse on the left. They sniff at one another. The horse on the left kicks with his left foreleg. ***Upper middle:*** The horse on the right turns around and threatens to kick. He does this by hopping backwards and threateningly lifting his hind legs up to his stomach. He does not actually kick backwards. ***Lower middle:*** He hops backwards without kicking. Pay attention to his face. The increased tension is clearly visible in his protruding upper lip and the pointed, cup-like shape of his lower lip. ***Bottom:*** Both horses walk to the back of the paddock. They start to graze, keeping their positions parallel to one another. There has been no conflict or injury, but there have been clear signals back and forth indicating how much space the horses need between each other.

3.13 BUCKING

Bucking is characterised by an expenditure of effort on the part of the horse. The back tenses, the neck is bent, the head is held low (underneath the chest or between the forelegs), and the horse jumps into the air with either both forelegs, both hind legs, or all four legs at once. As this happens, the hind legs may kick backwards. A horse may change direction as he bucks. Bucking can occur from a standstill, a walk, a trot, or a canter. A horse can buck for a long time with high intensity, or give a single buck with low intensity. When riding, if the rider keeps the horse's head up, he can also buck with a hollow back.

Bucking also occurs in play behaviour among horses. Unfortunately, I have very little video footage of this. I have, however, often observed bucking as a proactive behaviour to chase off a stimulus that is causing anxiety, pain, or fear (**Figs 3.65–3.67**). That is why I classify this signal as a distance increasing signal. The horse acts proactively to rid himself of a stimulus. I have seen the same motivation in horses at pasture. Bucking with hind leg kicking is used as a distance increasing signal in these situations. It is meant to warn others to keep their distance; therefore the kicks do not actually connect.

Bucking while being ridden may also be a proactive behaviour to stop a frustrating or painful stimulus, such as the rider, the equipment, or the riding commands being given. In this situation, the bucking may be accompanied by flight behaviour, ambivalent behaviour during which two behaviour systems are stimulated consecutively or at the same time.

For a rider, a horse who bucks while being ridden is generally frightening. It may also result in a dangerous situation for the horse, the rider, and any possible onlookers. Therefore, it is a good idea to find out if the bucking can be prevented. Pain may be the underlying cause, such as from an ill-fitting saddle, or if the rider is sitting in the saddle incorrectly. You should also try to find out if the horse is comfortable in the riding space and if he is not being asked to do too much, work-wise, which would build up tension he might then release by bucking. Bucking can become a learned mechanism if the result is positive for the horse.

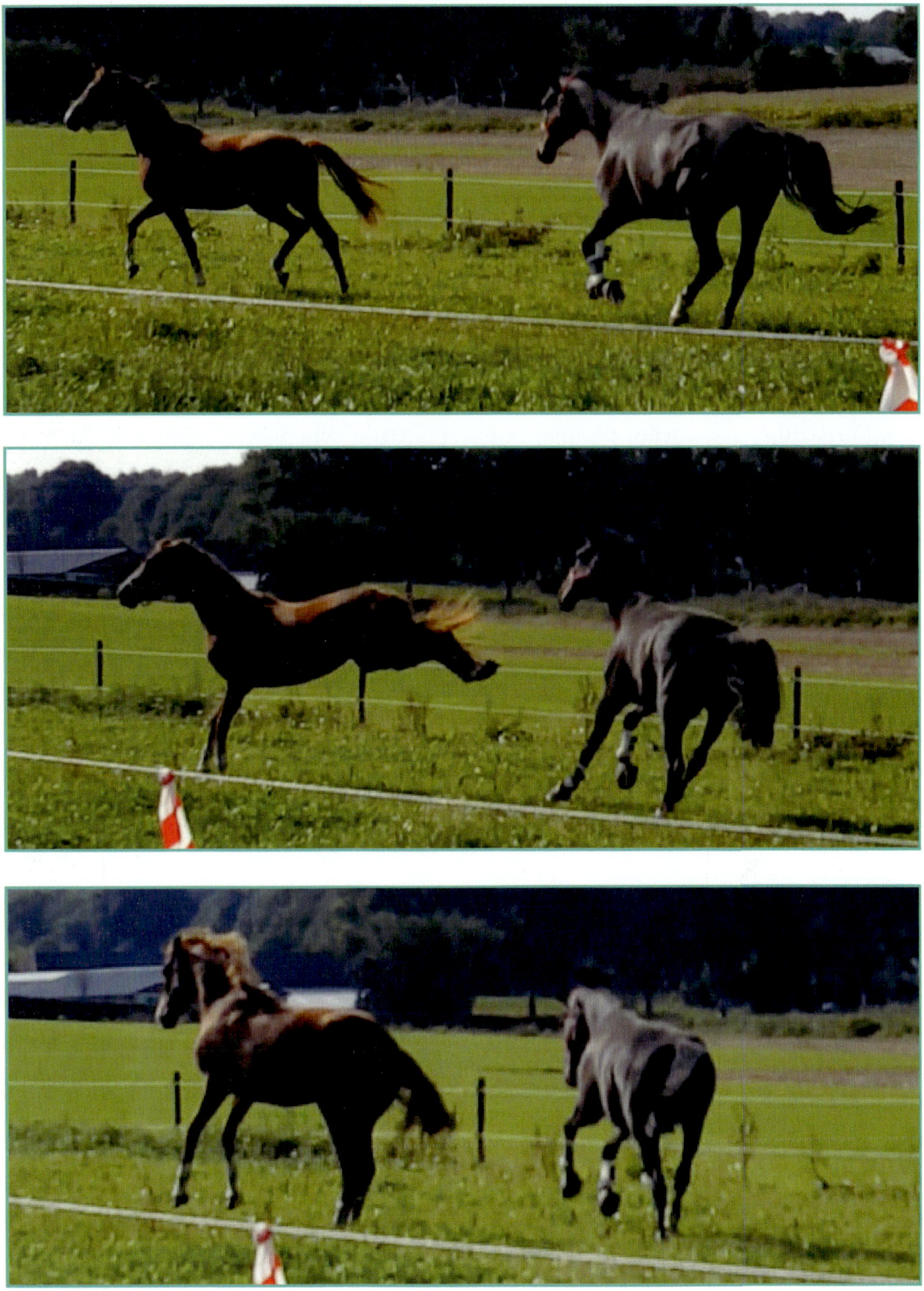

Figs 3.65–3.67 J'adore (the chestnut) and Gairo (the dark bay) are paired up and put into a paddock together for the first time. Both of them trot and canter towards the end of the paddock. Gairo comes too close to J'adore. She takes action by bucking to increase their distance. Gairo then moves away.

3.14 THE ARCHED NECK

The arched and tensed neck is a distance increasing signal during which a horse actively approaches the stimulus either in a straight line or at a curve. When the horse is passing or has just passed the stimulus, he may maintain the arched neck for several more seconds. The arched neck is characterised by a tensed and clearly visible splenius capitis muscle. The nose is also bent slightly towards the chest, arching the neck. The ears are mostly pointed forwards, but may also be turned back if the tension rises. I consider the arched neck to be a mild form of posturing behaviour (see section 3.15).

During my research, I have seen horses give this signal to people, animals, and objects that were unfamiliar to the horse, for example, when a horse out on a country ride passes an unfamiliar horse at pasture, when two horses who do not know each other are placed in the same paddock together, or when a horse is confronted with an unfamiliar object, person, or animal. The face of a horse who arches his neck clearly shows signs of high tension. In my research, the 'unfamiliar' horses, people, and objects reacted calmly to the signal and the encounter, without provoking the horse in any way, causing the tension of the horse with the arched neck to decrease very quickly (**Figs 3.68, 3.69**). The horse relaxed his neck almost immediately.

Also in my research, the arched neck occurred in horses who had been put into a certain situation. I can imagine that the horse, had he been free to choose, would have picked a different way to go about meeting a new stimulus. He might have avoided it entirely or positioned himself at a greater distance from the stimulus and taken much more time before actually making contact with it.

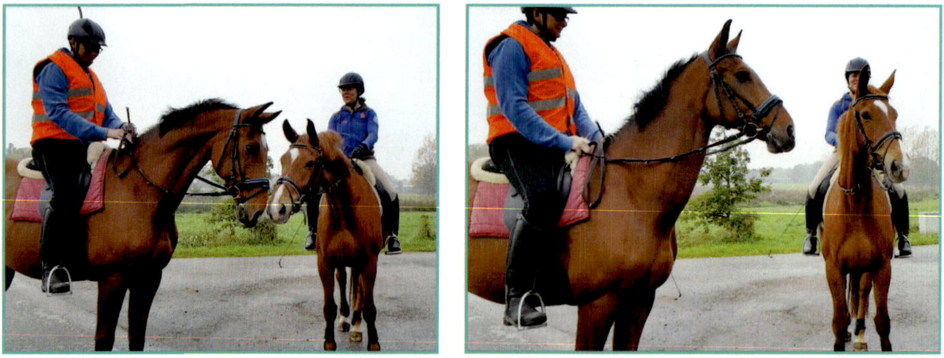

Fig. 3.68, 3.69 ***Left:*** Orion and Dana meet in the street. Orion is on the left, Dana on the right. They both have an arched neck, a distance increasing signal. But Dana also has another internal motivation: to meet Orion. She extends her nose to smell him. ***Right:*** The tension ebbs. The arched neck as a distance increasing signal disappears. Orion's facial features and tense muscles still reflect tension. Note that the reins on both horses are slack. No signals are being given by the riders.

In my observations, ninety-five percent of the time, the arched neck, just like other distance increasing signals, did not lead to confrontation and actual fighting (**Figs 3.70–3.75**). In the other five percent, however, the arched neck was followed by a foreleg kick (seriously aimed and connecting or not).

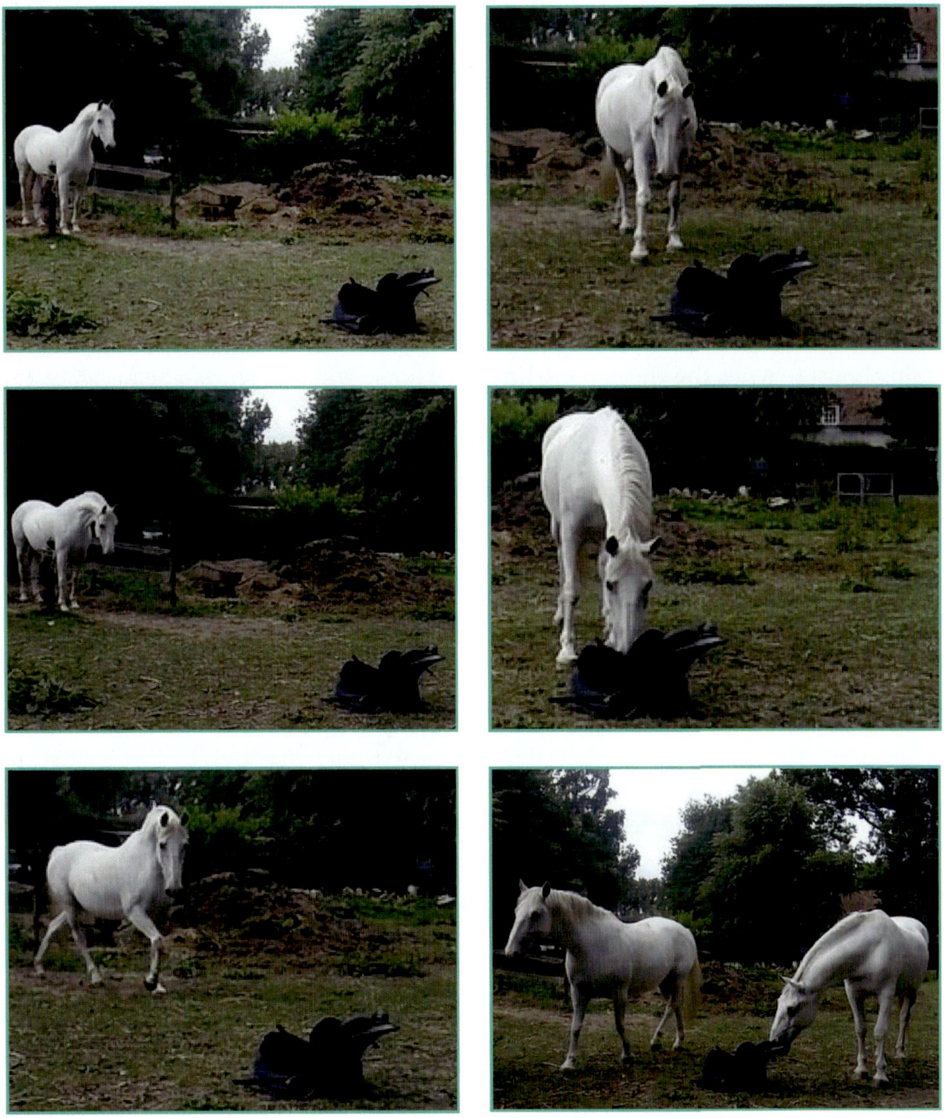

Figs 3.70–3.75 In the three photos on the left, you see Ilova approaching a saddle with an arched neck. She makes a shallow curve in her approach. In the three photos on the right, she examines the saddle. She finally walks away and another horse in the paddock takes over the investigation. On the video footage, when Ilova walks away you can see her chewing as a calming signal.

3.15 POSTURING BEHAVIOUR

Have you ever had to walk through a dark alley at night in a strange city? I have. And I have to say, I felt two conflicting impulses. One was a desire to run away as fast as I could (yes, out of fear), but because I saw no direct reason to be afraid and so could argue myself out of it, I calmly kept on walking. I straightened my back, squared my shoulders, and looked straight at anyone I saw. My vibes said, 'Don't mess with me!' Of course, I was totally relieved when I got to the end of the alley. Fair is fair.

While observing domesticated horses, I also encountered horses who showed posturing behaviour. In this study I mostly witnessed them doing so when they saw new horses, so the other horse was the direct cause of the posturing behaviour. The attention of the horse who displays the posturing behaviour is also completely focused on the other horse. He makes himself much bigger. It even seems as if his body is being inflated or pumped up a bit. The muscle tension increases. The neck arches (see section 3.14), the ears point forward, and the head is bent so that the chin almost touches the chest. Sometimes the horse will also show a head swing. He makes dancing, high-stepping paces. The tail is carried light to high, high, or very high, in which case the tail may stick up vertically. During this posturing behaviour, the horse may have loud, snort-like breathing and also expel a hard puff of air.

The posturing behaviour I mostly saw during my research happened between horses who had not met yet and passed each other at a distance in different ways. It could have been when one horse was at pasture and the other passed by, or when two horses passed each other in the woods during a ride. It almost never came to an actual meeting between these horses. The owners kept them at a distance, because a meeting had not been planned. I categorise the posturing behaviour horses show under these circumstances as distance increasing behaviour. By displaying posturing behaviour, the horse seems to intimidate the other horse so much that it prevents escalation. Horses who were intimidated responded to this behaviour by giving calming signals. They did not provoke the horse who was intimidating them, and so matters did not escalate. If the horse who was displaying the posturing behaviour passed by the other horse, or stood parallel to the other horse (so with his flank facing him) at great distance, then the tension level dropped, the posturing behaviour abated, and the horse started moving again in the same way as before the posturing behaviour.

The key to handling this type of behaviour is, I think, maintaining distance until the horse feels comfortable with the other animal, even if this takes a few encounters to accomplish. Getting angry at your horse for acting independently from you towards other horses forces him to deal with additional negative associations, and maybe even pain, on top of an already tense situation.

The four horses in **Figs 3.76–3.78** are first-time neighbours in a paddock.

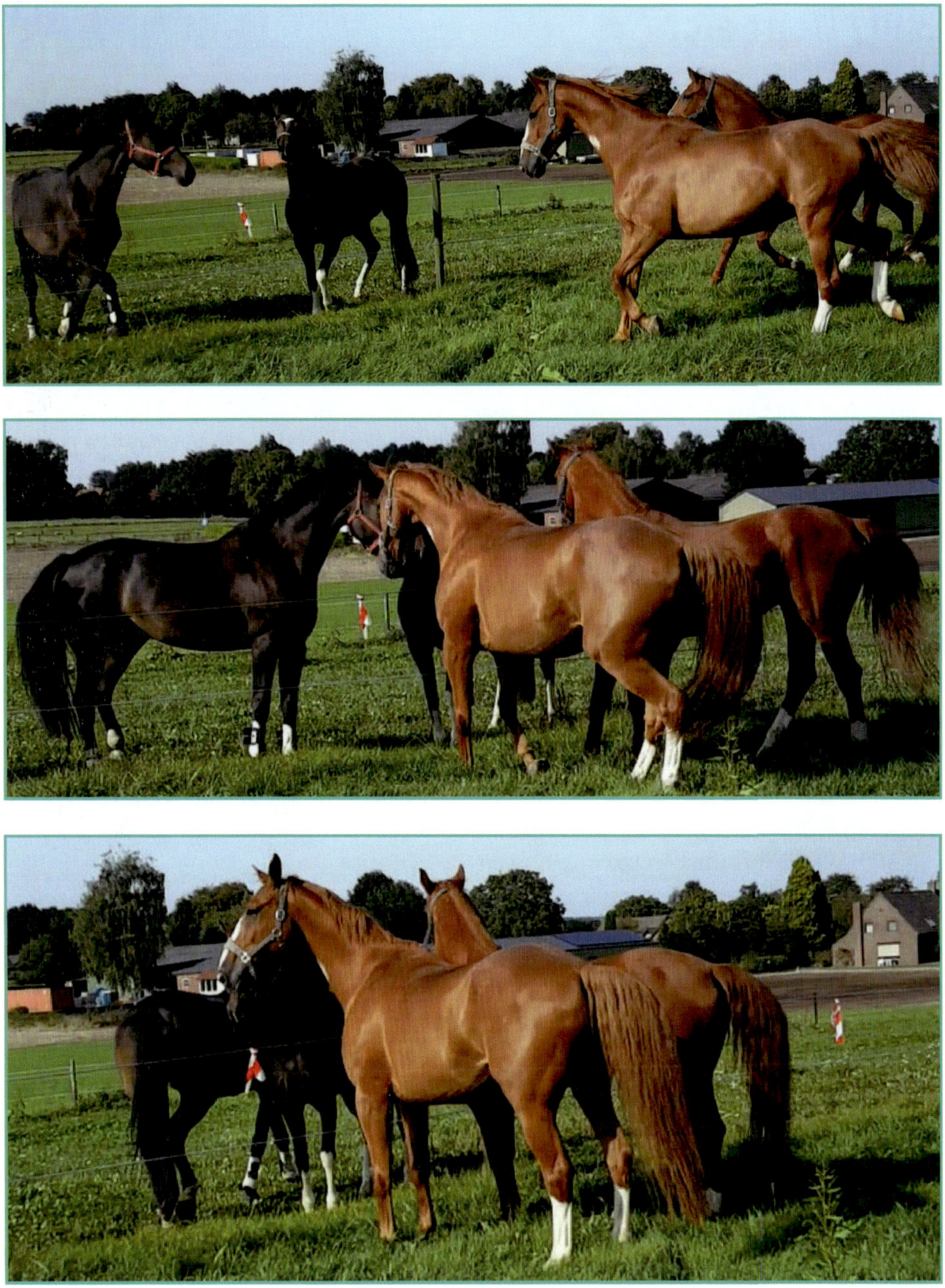

Figs 3.76–3.78 ***Top:*** Vosje, the chestnut at the front left of the photo is frontally approaching Gairo, the dark bay horse on the left and the only other gelding. Vosje has an arched neck and trots in a way that indicates posturing behaviour. It is a distance increasing signal towards Gairo. ***Middle:*** Gairo responds with an arched neck. The horses sniff at each other. ***Bottom:*** Gairo does not want to incite conflict. He walks away.

3.16 FLIGHT SIGNALS

Fleeing is a distance increasing signal in which the horse moves away from the disturbing stimulus. Flight behaviour can occur at different levels of intensity, the size of the flight behaviour being proportional to how much tension the horse is feeling (and showing through associated body features): a weakened form of fleeing in cases of light tension (**Fig. 3.79**) and intense flight behaviour in cases of high tension (**Fig. 3.80**).

An example of a weakened form of fleeing is, for example, when a horse who is tied up steps away from a rider who is trying to hose him down after riding. A flight reaction with medium tension could be when a horse at pasture is startled by a sound and trots away from it. A flight reaction with high tension could be when a horse who is afraid to leave home is on a ride in the woods and turns around to flee back to the stable. It is obvious that every horse has his own associations with the world around him. In the same way, every horse has his own plethora of tensions and fears.

Typical features of flight behaviour are:

1 Ears that are turned back if the horse intends to flee and when he actually flees (before the horse turns his ears back, he may rotate them very carefully in order to catch sounds from as many directions as possible). During the flight, the ears may alternate to a forward position towards the direction the horse is heading.
2 The horse holding his head up, extending his nose, and forming a hollow back.
3 A tail that is always tense. This may indicate a mild, medium, or high tension. A relaxed tail is impossible in a horse who is fleeing.
4 A head that is turned slightly sideways for a moment, allowing the horse to see the object he is turning away from. If the horse is fleeing, both ears will turn forwards, in the direction the horse is going.

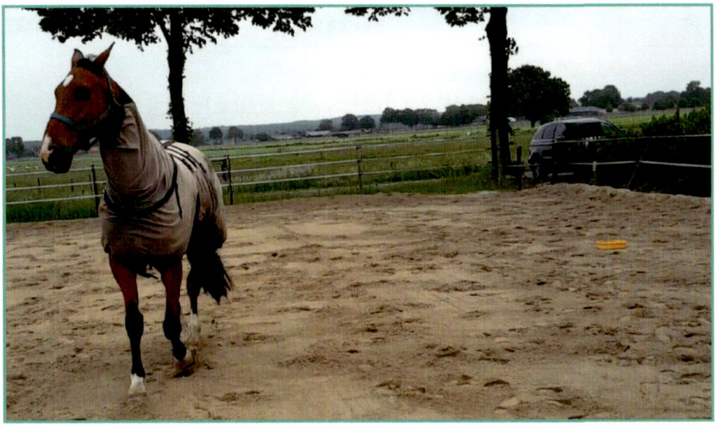

Fig. 3.79 Orion is afraid of the back-right corner of the arena. He walks away from it, showing flight behaviour with light tension.

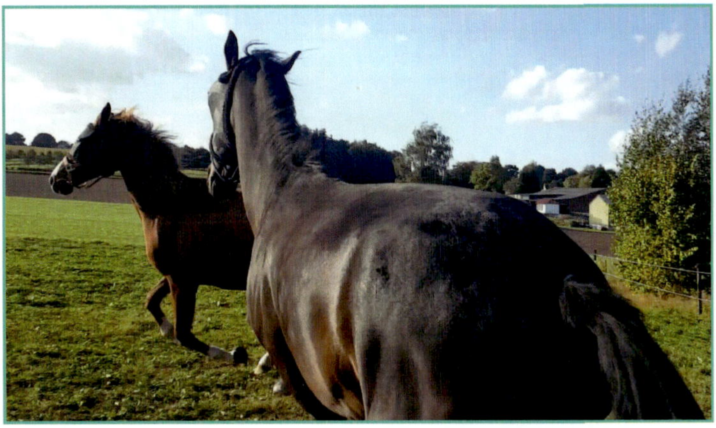

Fig. 3.80 Both horses are startled near the paddock gate. In the blink of an eye, they turn and sprint off. At the start of the flight they hold their ears back. Then both ears will turn forwards in the direction the horses are heading.

3.17 EXAMPLE OF A BEHAVIOUR SEQUENCE

In the following series of photos (**Figs 3.81–3.93**) you can see splitting and distance increasing signals of fleeing and taking action. The situation: the smaller chestnut Lorain is a valuable possession. The larger chestnut Vosje, and the spotted horse, Saar, both want to be with her. Saar makes an attempt at this.

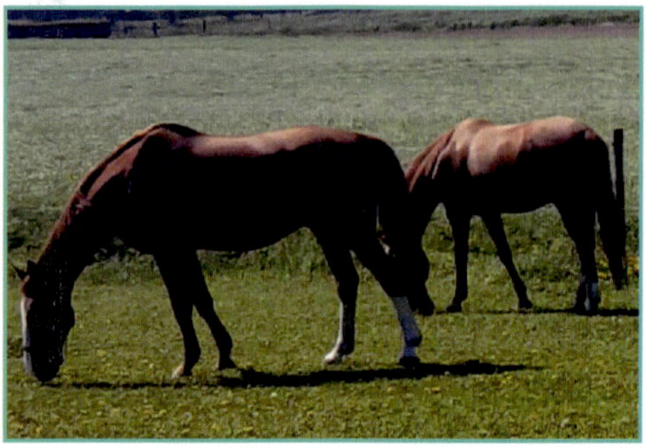

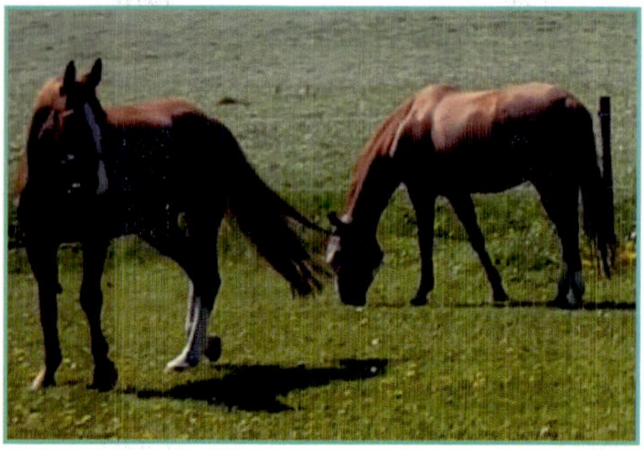

Figs 3.81, 3.82 Vosje and Lorain are grazing. Vosje sees Saar approaching in a straight line.

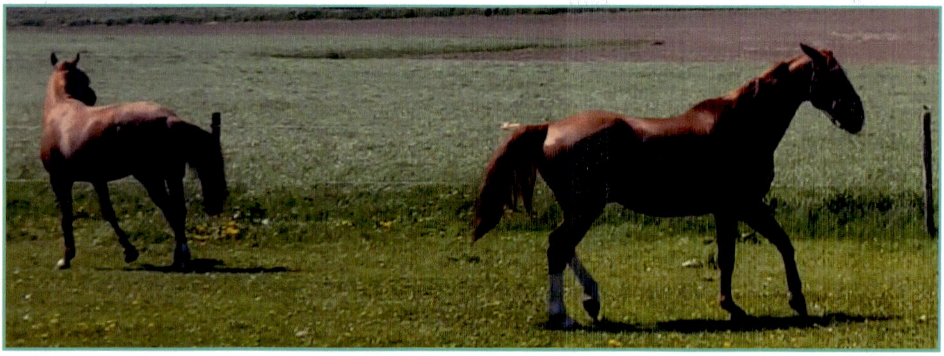

Fig. 3.83 Vosje chases Saar (who is not yet in the photo) away. This is a distance increasing signal.

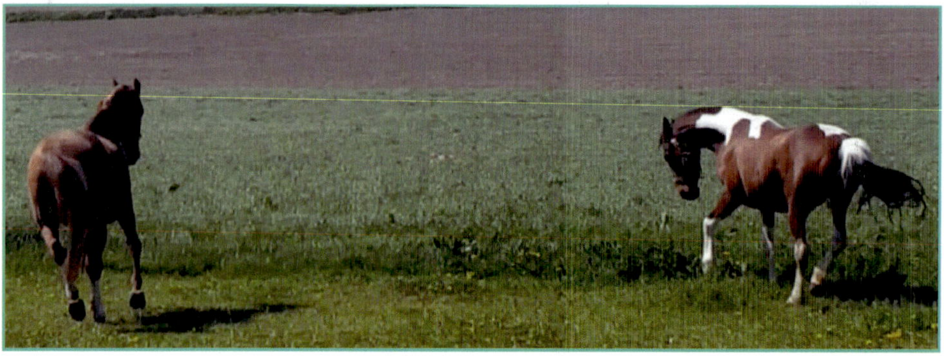

Fig. 3.84 Saar drives Vosje away. Vosje does not flee. He chases Saar away and splits between her and Lorain, who is to his left.

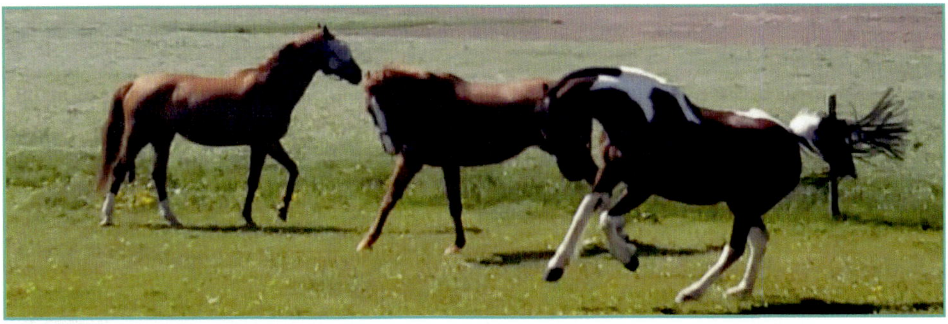

Fig. 3.85 Saar bends to the left. Vosje keeps chasing her away and splits between her and Lorain. Saar also has a chasing off posture.

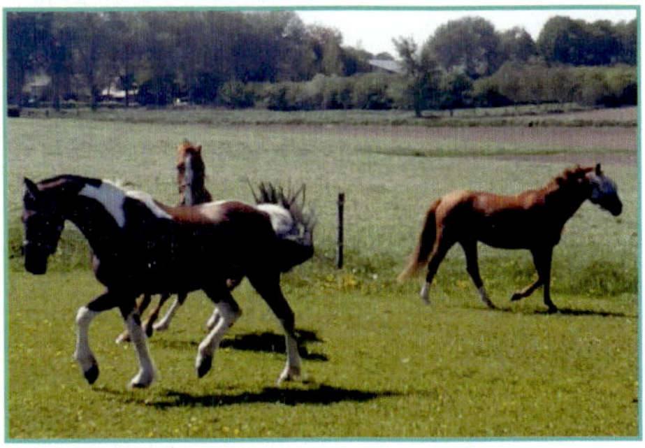

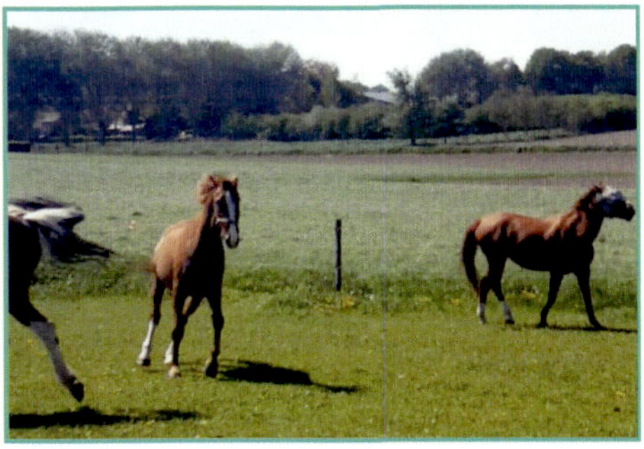

Figs 3.86, 3.87 Saar increases the distance by fleeing. Vosje drives her away.

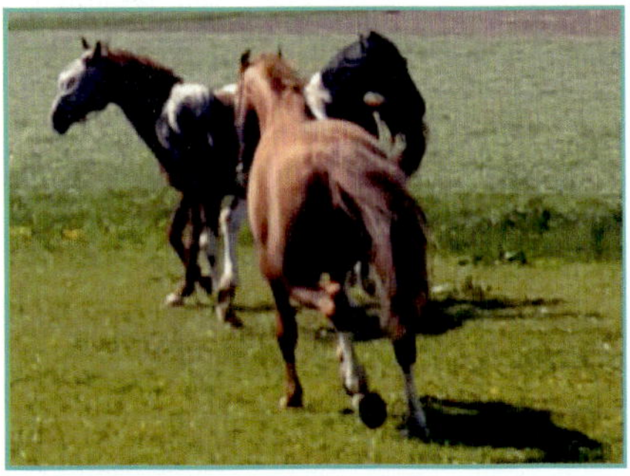

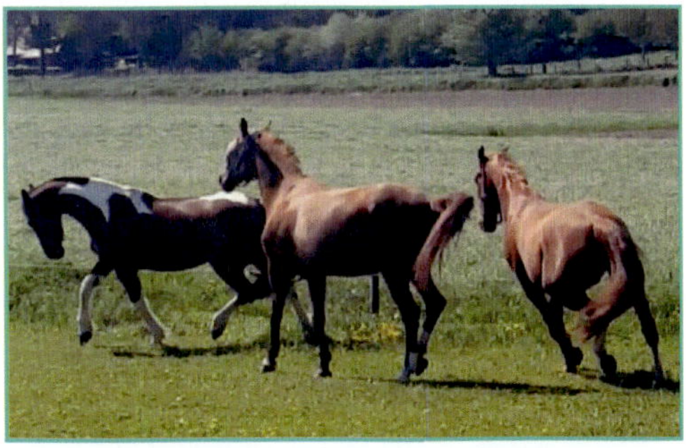

Figs 3.88, 3.89 As Vosje canters in an arc, Saar turns around to canter around Lorain. Vosje chases Saar away.

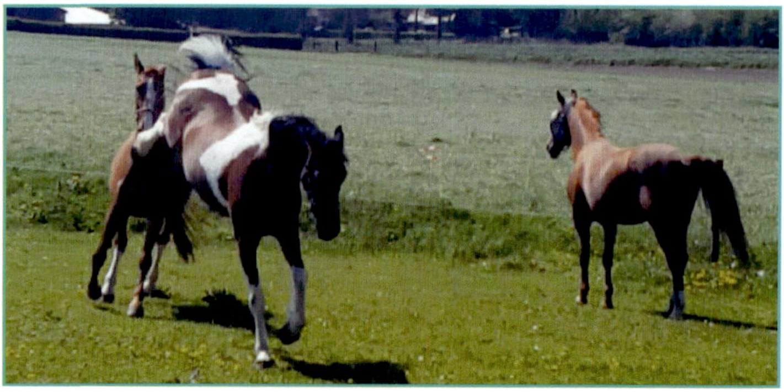

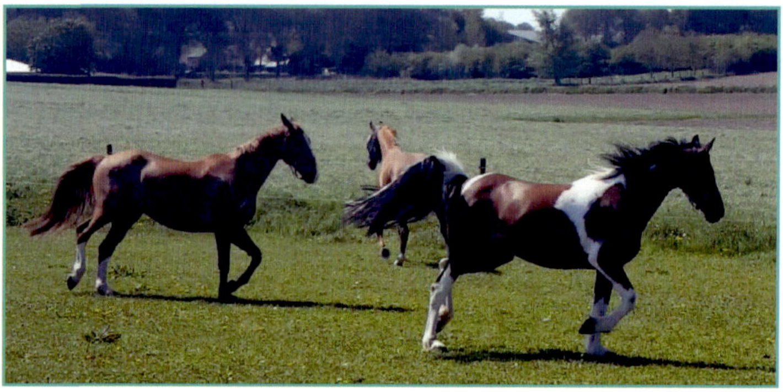

Figs 3.90, 3.91 Vosje keeps chasing Saar away. She flees and gives an added distance increasing signal: she bucks and kicks with her hind legs, but does not connect with Vosje. Vosje drives Saar away, at the same time turning left to split up Saar and Lorain. Saar's ears are pointed to where she is going: forwards. Her high tail shows lingering tension.

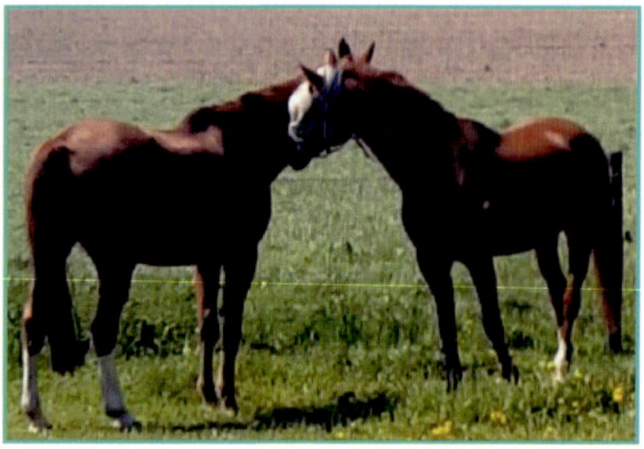

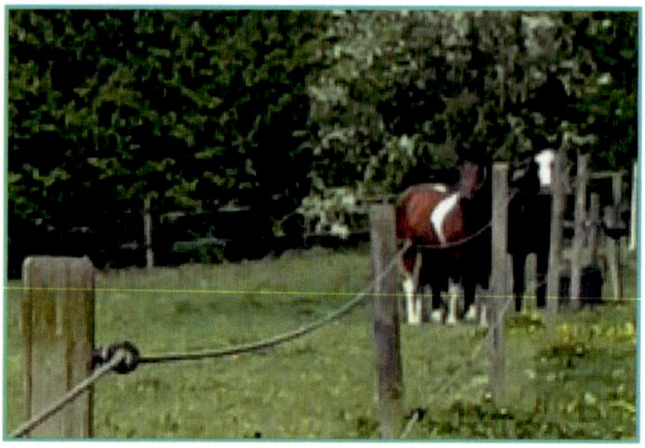

Figs 3.92, 3.93 All's well that ends well? Vosje and Lorain are together, with Saar and Oscar looking on from a great distance.

3.18 FIGHT OR FLIGHT

If the type of tension we have been discussing in previous sections in this chapter does not decrease, and if the distance increasing signals are not lowering the tension, the signals will become stronger and the horse will start to take real action. At this point, we are talking about fight or flight. Not threatening to kick, but actually purposefully hitting the other horse with a foreleg or hind leg. Not threatening to bite, but really biting. Not calmly walking or trotting away, but running as if his life depended on it. In this situation, there is no bucking as the horse runs; he uses all his energy to flee the situation or, possibly, he kicks as he runs in order to fend off an attacker.

Freezing is another response you can come across on this spectrum. This is different from the calming signal of immobility. Freezing is characterised by a body that is stiff with tension. The horse assumes the highest head–neck position and both the eyes and the nostrils can be very round. Sometimes you can see or feel the horse's heartbeat. One of his legs may tremble.

From my observations the moment of freezing is something that can happen just before a fight or flight response. It is a moment of very tense immobility, followed by an actual fight or flight reaction.

There are no more calming signals or displacement behaviour to be seen. When the tension is this high, the horse no longer eats, drinks, or defecates. These activities only resume when the peak of the tension has dropped and the tension starts to decrease generally.

I have observed a number of the horses featured in this research under different circumstances, both during their association with people and as they interacted with other horses at pasture. What I noticed was that when a few of these horses experienced increasing tension, they expressed it differently with people than with other horses.

When experiencing increasing tension while around people, these horses showed stress signals, stress behaviours and distance increasing signals. It did not lead to a fight response, such as an actual bite or kick directed at people, or if it did, the response came in an extremely weakened form. However, when these horses were at pasture, they did show fight responses towards other horses.

This fight response could be very varied in intensity and underlying tension, ranging from a softer connecting kick to a harder strike. Alternatively, one horse would bite another softly, although still leaving a mark in the coat or a hairless spot, or harder, causing a scratch or, with an even higher intensity and motivation, a deeper injury.

If the horse showed a lower intensity fight response in reaction to another horse, it would have been preceded by less build-up of tension. I have not observed displacement behaviours in these situations. The amount of time in which the horse showed distance increasing signals could also vary greatly.

These might be given hardly at all, or not at all, or given for a longer time before a fight response followed.

Of course it is difficult to compare different situations, and one must draw conclusions from such comparisons with the greatest care, especially because every horse has his own internal motivation for what he finds important and brings his own baggage when it comes to the things he has learned and experienced in his life. Also, the horse may be in a different mood from one situation to another. However, I do want to suggest, on the basis of my observations, that for some horses the threshold for committing violence seems lower in relation to other horses than to people, as well as producing less prolonged stress in advance. It seems very plausible to me that this is because people teach horses not to give physical fight responses. We do not allow horses to bite or kick with the foreleg or hind leg. It makes sense that this may cause the horse to experience elevated stress for longer in what is for him a difficult situation, and that it has a strong effect on his behaviour and communication signals in his interaction with people.

On the internet, there is footage of horses who, apparently out of nowhere, show an extremely strong fight response towards people; for example, a kick or bite at full force. Usually, these videos are edited to show the actual moment of biting or kicking over and over again. What happens before then is not shown. You need to see this in order to assess an element of behaviour in a behavioural sequence, and also to judge if the horse is showing signs of tension. In my research I have always seen these signs. They may have developed over a long time or rise to the fore quickly when a situation arises out of nowhere. Never in my research have I observed a fight response directed at people without seeing tension features or distance increasing signals first. But is it possible? Perhaps, if the horse has internalised a fight response, such as biting or kicking at full force, as an entirely normal means of communication and coping mechanism in his life, so that it is not preceded by an obvious increase of tension (including the associated behaviours).

WHAT IS LEARNING?

At what point a horse shows this freezing and fight or flight mechanism depends on the severity of the stimulus, the horse himself, his nature, his life experiences, or his bond with his rider. Some horses show two calming signals, one displacement behaviour, five stress signals, and then flee. Others will, in the same situation, show as many as 10 calming signals and five stress signals before they flee. Some horses may only show stress signals. Sometimes there can be minutes between a stimulus and a fight or flight mechanism, sometimes only a split second, such as when a horse is startled by a stimulus (discussed in section 3.20).

When a horse freezes, fights, or flees, he is operating under a primordial drive to react and survive. Learning is almost impossible. But what type of learning are we talking about? Recognising the connection between the emotion of fear and an associated stimulus (for a horse this is a very useful skill needed for survival purposes), or learning to obey us, to control himself because we feel that the situation or stimulus is fine and believe that the horse ought to understand that it is not scary?

In my experience, a horse remembers a stimulus that has caused fear or even a fight or flight response very well, and if he has not overcome this fear by himself, or not has been desensitised or habituated to it, he will naturally keep responding more fearfully to it in the future. Not only that, but as time goes by a generalisation of the stimulus can occur whereby the horse starts to react with fear or suspicion not only to the original stimulus, but also to stimuli that are similar or to circumstances such as those present when he was first frightened (a location, a sound, etc).

It is difficult to say to what extent a horse can still reason and follow along in our thinking and learn to behave in the way we want him to in a situation of increasing tension. It will depend on various factors. Here are a few examples:

- The more relaxed the learning climate, the better the horse will be able to concentrate on cognitive tasks and the better he will be able to control himself should the need arise.
- The better an exercise is built up, step by step, the easier it is for the horse to follow along and remember.
- The more our solution and modus operandi suits the nature and internal motivation of the horse, the more easily he will pick it up.
- The more sense our request makes to the horse, the more easily he will pick it up.
- The better socialised he is, the better his brain structure will be in terms of working neurons and synapses, providing him with the kind of brain structure that can support thinking and reasoning, resulting in fewer fight or flight responses on his part.
- The better socialised he is, the more easily he will associate new stimuli with already formed, cognitively established concepts in his brain.
- The more the horse is used to appealing to his own cognitive abilities and reasoning, the better his problem solving skills will be and the less likely he will be to show instinctive fight or flight responses.

In my opinion, if a rider or handler interprets his horse's body signals more precisely, makes sure to recognise calming signals, and adapts the learning circumstances in order to avoid high tension, he will be dealing with a horse who feels better, learns and remembers more easily, and therefore requires less time and repetition in learning certain exercises. This mainly happens when a horse is mentally and physically healthy.

3.19 COMMUNICATION LADDER: FIGHT OR FLIGHT

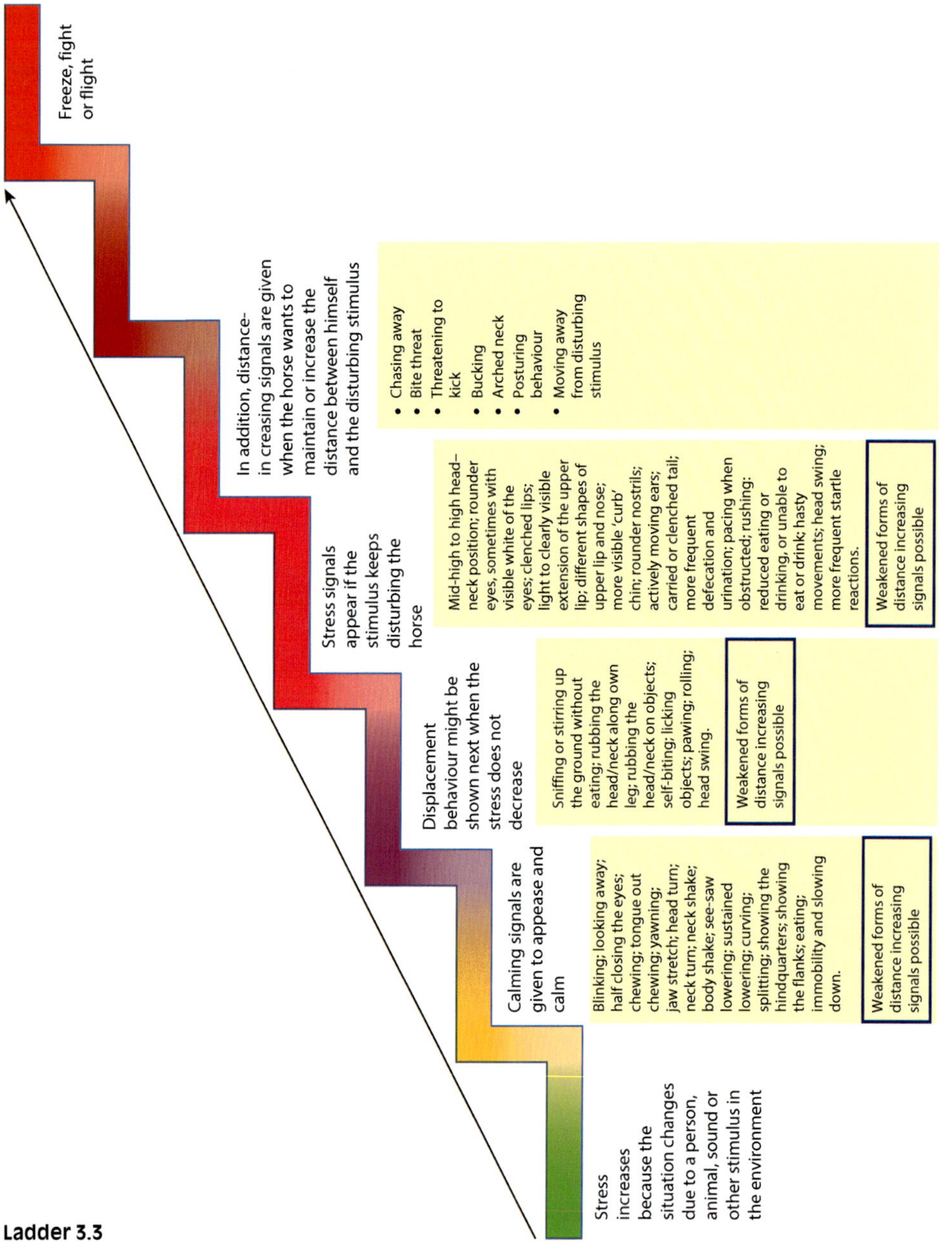

Ladder 3.3

3.20 RECOVERY AFTER MOUNTING TENSION AND SHOCK

In the previous sections we discussed tension continuously increasing until the horse shows a fight or flight response. However, when you deal with horses you will also come across situations in which there is no or hardly any gradual increase in tension. This happens when the horse is suddenly confronted by a new stimulus that comes out of nowhere, or a reaction to an existing stimulus, that causes him to feel mild to severe shock, including all the tension features and behaviours that go with this. Where there is a sudden shock, the same underlying biological processes as previously described in this chapter take place.

I am riding Vosje in the woods. It is May. The weather is beautiful and pale sunshine dapples through the trees. We are trotting along a long, straight path. To the side of the path is a dense thicket. Suddenly, Vosje's trot changes. He makes himself much bigger. His paces become shorter and higher. His head goes straight up into the air. His nostrils are round and he is snorting. His eyes are round, and he carries his tail high (yes, I sometimes awkwardly turn on my horse to look back and see). I see nothing that may explain his behaviour. I slow him to a walk. Vosje's head–neck position remains very high and his ears and eyes stay round. He dances with high-stepping paces, his tail held very high. He sometimes emits a hard snorting noise. Forty metres away, I see a deer in the thicket. After we pass him, Vosje slows down. His tails lowers a little, as does his head–neck position. He shows a see-saw lowering a couple of times. He chews and his nostrils go from round to long.

When you look at how a horse recovers from a fight or flight response or a strong or mild shock, you will see that the elements that form the upward communication ladder also feature on the downward ladder. The same steps are taken, for which the following applies:

1 The position on the communication ladder depends on the intensity of the shock. The biggest shock causes an immediate fight or flight response. A large shock causes tension, and the horse may or may not show distance increasing signals. A lighter shock is recovered from more quickly, after which displacement behaviour or calming signals can be seen. How long a horse takes to recover from a shock depends on the severity of the stimulus, the horse's life experiences, and his physical and mental condition at that time.
2 When a horse is recovering from a shock and the process has not fully finished, you will see that his threshold for responding to stimuli is lower. He will more easily be startled by stimuli he would normally be able to handle.

3 Every horse uses his own signals from within the communication groups. One horse will use multiple signals from a communication group consecutively or simultaneously, while another will use only one or two.
4 The ability to actually give the signals also plays a role here. A horse who is at pasture and is startled will use rolling as a displacement behaviour more quickly because he can easily do so there, while a horse who is being ridden is not able to do this. This horse may, for instance, be more inclined to rub his head along his foreleg or show a see-saw lowering.
5 The displacement activities and calming signals form the last steps on the way down to relaxation. They allow the last of the tension to trickle away.

3.21 COMMUNICATION LADDER: RECOVERY AFTER TENSION AND SHOCK

Ladder 3.4

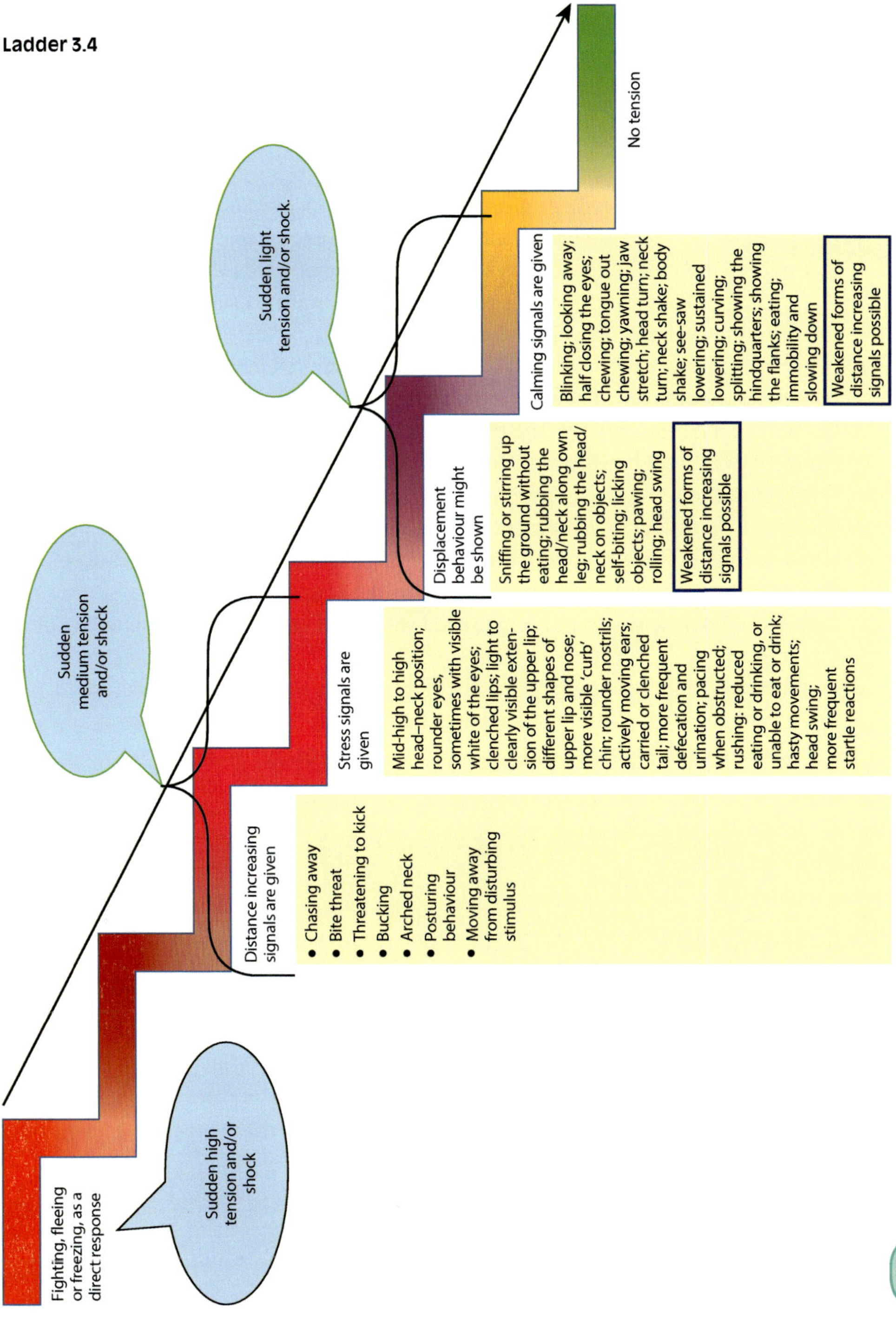

3.22 SUMMARY: RISING TENSION AND RECOVERY

- It is necessary to offer new stimuli in order to maintain cell renewal and brain plasticity. This keeps the horse mentally fit. A well-planned offering of stimuli also improves the horse's socialisation and his understanding of the world around him. Too many stimuli that the horse cannot handle lead to incidental stress. Cognitive abilities diminish during high incidental stress. If incidental stress occurs often, it can lead to chronic stress.
- Chronic stress causes cell deterioration in the hippocampus, which leads to deterioration of the cognitive abilities, memory capacity, and impulse control. It results in increased cell activity in the amygdala and this leads to an increased fear and aggression response. Chronic stress can in time cause a weakening of the immune system and depression.
- A horse experiences tension due to increasing stimulus intensity or startle responses that may or may not be predictable. The basic features of a tense horse are that as the tension rises, the horse starts to hold his head and neck between a mid-high and high position. There is also muscle tension throughout the body. The higher the tension, the rounder the eyes and nostrils become. The mouth shows the following development when there is tension: tense lips, clenched lips, and possibly an extension of the upper lip or differently shaped lip and nose. The chin is tensed, forming a more square, cup-like shape. The tail may assume a number of positions, from lightly carried to carried vertically or clenched against the anus.
- In situations of increasing tension, the horse wants to increase the distance from the stimulus that is causing the tension. He may do this by moving away from the stimulus and fleeing or by taking action against the disturbing stimulus, such as chasing it away, threatening to bite or kick, arching his neck, or showing posturing behaviour. The goal of this is to not engage in actual fighting or inflict or incur injury. If the object does not respond adequately, or if the stimulus intensity increases, the horse may actually fight or flee.
- The more intense the shock or fight or flight response, the longer the horse's recovery will take.

3.23 REFERENCES

1 McEwen BS (2004) Protection and damage from acute and chronic stress: allostasis and allostatic overload and relevance to the pathophysiology of psychiatric disorders. *Ann N Y Acad Sci* **1032:**1–7.

2 National Scientific Council on the Developing Child (2014) *Excessive Stress Disrupts the Architecture of the Developing Brain: Working Paper 3*. Updated Edition. http://developingchild.harvard.edu/resources/wp3/

3 Panksepp J, Biven L (2012) *The Archaeology of Mind. Neuroevolutionary Origins of Human Emotions*. W.W. Norton & Company, New York, p. 335.

4 Nyberg J (2014) *The Adaptable Brain*. Lecture at The Dog Symposium, Oslo.

5 Panksepp J, Biven L (2012) *The Archaeology of Mind. Neuroevolutionary Origins of Human Emotions*. W.W. Norton & Company, New York, p. 176.

6 Cooper J, McGreevy P (2003) Stereotypic behaviour in the stabled horse: causes, effects and prevention without compromising horse welfare. In: *The Welfare of Horses*. (ed. N Waran) Kluwer Academic Publishers, Dordrecht, pp. 99–124.

7 McGreevy P, McLean A (2010) *Equitation Science*. Wiley-Blackwell, Ames, p. 231.

8 Sapolsky RM (2004) *Why Zebras Don't Get Ulcers. The Acclaimed Guide to Stress, Stress-Related Diseases, and Coping*, 3rd edn. St Martin's Griffin, New York, p. 221.

9 McGreevy P, McLean A (2010) *Equitation Science*. Wiley-Blackwell, Ames, p. 228.

10 Mertz H, UNC Center for Functional GI and Motility Disorders. *Stress and the Gut*. http://www.med.unc.edu/ibs/files/educational-gi-handouts/Stress%20and%20the%20Gut.pdf

11 Patra PB, Patra S (2015) Research findings on overactive bladder. *Curr Urol* **8:**1–21.

4 *No communication*

MY RESEARCH has shone light on horses' communication signals. In the previous chapters I have described the range of communication signals that horses use. However, I have also come across situations in which horses do not communicate. This can be for a number of reasons, listed below, which will be discussed more extensively in this chapter:

- The horses were not interested in me or in possible communication.
- The horses required no communication. They were able to handle the situation on their own.
- Learned habits have taken the place of communication signals.
- The horse was hindered in his attempt to communicate.
- It was a case of withdrawal and stereotyped behaviour.

4.1 JUST NOT THAT INTERESTED

Communication is a process in which you make contact with yourself, your environment, or elements in your environment, living or inanimate. However, horses do not respond to every stimulus in their environment. It will depend on the horse and the situation, on what the horse has learned throughout his life, and on what he can handle. So when does a horse not respond to stimuli?

WHEN THESE ARE SO NORMAL FOR HIM THAT HE DOES NOT NEED TO RESPOND

This is something you will see, for example, in a horse who has for years been occupying a paddock that is bordered by a walking path. The horse will have seen so many different people, people in all shapes and sizes, pass by over the years that he no longer responds to a new person. He just keeps grazing. If he does look, it is with a totally relaxed expression: a mid-high head–neck position, ears pointed forwards, almond-shaped eyes, long nostrils, and a relaxed mouth in which the lower lip is also relaxed and perhaps protrudes in front of the upper lip a little. There are no tight lines in the face or body and no tense muscles.

You will also see this, for example, in a horse who is being saddled and has no problem with this at all. He stands still, relaxed. He moves an ear around, following the rider, but he is also looking around. His head is relaxed, with soft, almond-shaped eyes, long nostrils, relaxed lips.

YOU WOULD NOT RESPOND TO A STIMULUS THAT DOES NOT INTEREST YOU EITHER

In this situation, you would choose to just go your own way without reacting. This could happen, for example, if your horse has just been put out into a paddock with fresh, long grass. He starts to eat, sees or hears a stimulus, but chooses not to look or respond in some other way but just keeps on grazing. Of course, these are stimuli that the horse can handle or that only stimulate him very mildly. If he is grazing and something happens that is outside of his comfort zone, he will react.

People can experience this as well. When you are sitting at a pavement café with a friend, you do not communicate with passers-by and the passers-by do not communicate with you, maintaining a stress-free situation. In this situation both parties do not seek to be in contact with or elicit communication with each other.

When the situation or the object does not prompt communication

This is shown in diagrammatic form in the communication ladder in the next section.

4.2 COMMUNICATION LADDER: NO COMMUNICATION SIGNALS

Ladder 4.1

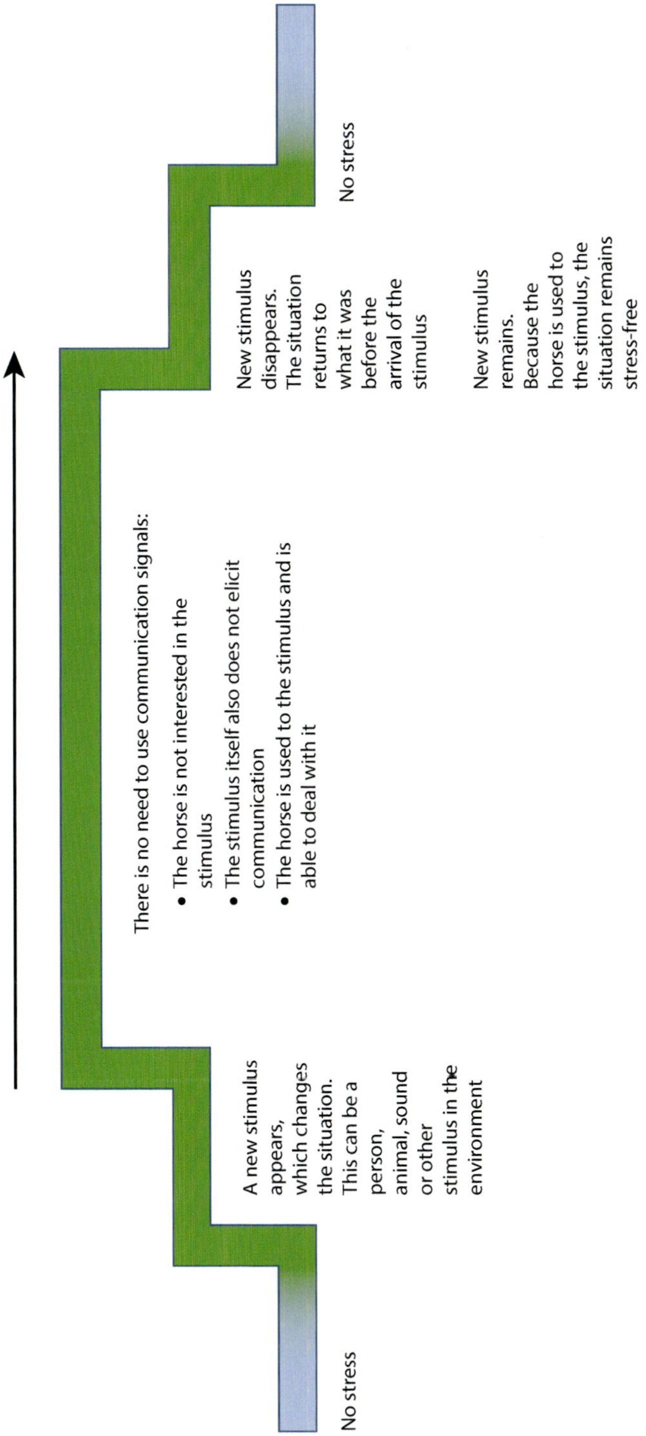

LEARNED HABIT

There are a number of other situations in which the horse does not show natural communication when in connection with people. This is the case, for instance, when a learned habit has replaced natural communication signals. The horse may have taught himself this learned habit because he has found the outcome of the behaviour to be rewarding, or the handler may have taught the horse a trick that replaced the natural behaviour. An example of this might be:

After being ridden, the horse is given feed in his trough. However, his owner first makes him lift a foreleg, as if giving a paw. When the horse does this, he gets his feed. After some time has passed, the horse understands this. He will stand with his foreleg up in the air until he gets his feed. When this takes too long, he may put his foreleg down, lift it again, and keep repeating the exercise. In this situation, the learned behaviour (and possibly the associated stress) has replaced, or alternates with, the expression of natural communication, although any possible stress signals given when the feed is not immediately offered are also natural communication signals.

IMPEDIMENT TO COMMUNICATION

When horses are accompanied by people, it is possible that the people hinder them from showing communication signals, especially when they are being ridden. Riders may stop their horse from lowering the head or doing a head turn or a neck turn.

When a horse wants to carefully approach an unknown object, he may turn his hindquarters towards it first, then turn his flank towards it, and finally walk towards it in a curve, possibly pausing a couple of times along the way. This tactic is totally different from that of the rider, who often steers the horse straight towards the object. This may cause a disruption in communication. The horse is not ready to approach the object head-on, which increases his fear and may even result in a flight response.

4.3 WITHDRAWAL AND STEREOTYPED BEHAVIOUR

SHUTTING DOWN AND WITHDRAWING

Another group of horses who no longer communicate or respond to stimuli from the environment are horses who seem to withdraw into themselves and completely shut down in reaction to a stimulus. This can happen when the stimulus has just occurred, but it can also happen that a horse goes into shut-down mode under certain circumstances or while doing a particular activity due to bad experiences in the past. In this situation, the shut down is not a direct response to a stimulus that is present now, but it has become a habit in response to a stimulus that they were not able to handle in the past and after which they have developed the coping mechanism that they still use, even if the stimulus that provoked it is long gone.

When standing still during an extreme shut down, a horse's head is held in the horizontal, mid-low, or low position. His eyes are half closed. His ears can be in any position, but generally they are turned a little to the side or back. These eye and ear positions are held for a variable time without change or movement. There is very little facial expression when it comes to tensing of the chin, mouth, and nose. The horse does not respond to stimuli from the environment at all, or he hardly responds, or his response is delayed.

This body posture may remind you of a horse who is asleep or dozing, and it may be that your horse is indeed doing this. Take your time to have a good look and compare your horse with relaxed horses in similar situations who are able to handle stimuli in their environment. These horses look at the world in a relaxed way, as if they are watching television. They are in contact with the world around them. They have a horizontal to mid-high head–neck position, they look around, and move their ears in accordance with the situation. There seems to be a healthy balance between enjoyment of, and engagement with, life and they are able to handle what is asked of them and how they live.

NOT STANDING ON THEIR OWN FEET

It is important that horses who shut down from stimuli like this are recognised as such; this can be overlooked by riders because these horses seem calm and obedient.

Because these horses are very often not taught to deal with the stimulus they find difficult to cope with, or because they have been punished in the past for taking action, they remain dependent on their rider or handler to get them out of the situation and basically lack their own coping mechanism for handling the situation in a relaxed manner. Even when they are becoming stressed and, if they can take action to change the situation to their benefit, they will not do so. In this situation, the term 'learned helplessness' applies.

Learned helplessness is when an animal learns to be passive in response to a stressful situation. At first, these animals do show attempts to communicate or flee the situation. In my observations – observations that fell outside the scope of this research study – the horses have high tension and use strong communication signals.

However, because their behaviour has no effect and the animal cannot escape the stressful circumstances, they learn to be passive. If, later on, they encounter a stressful situation from which they *are* able to escape, a majority will no longer do so.[1,2] The passivity has become ingrained. In my observations there is variation in the degree to which a horse, in time, gives signals before he then shuts down. Some horses show a lot of stress signals; others first show small calming signals or extremely weakened fight or flight responses before they go into shut down. Depending on the intensity of the stimulus, the duration of the stimulus, the horse's health at the time, and his experiences in life, the shut down can last for a longer or shorter time.

Learned helplessness also happens through flooding. This is a form of applied therapy in which people or animals are bombarded or 'flooded' with the stimulus that is causing fear. This stimulus is permanently present at full strength, and there is no way to escape it. In people, flooding can be a successful form of therapy. It helps people to get used to the previously frightening stimulus because, through experience, they come to see that it is not as dangerous as they had imagined. Doing exactly the same with animals, however, is not a good idea. In my opinion there is a big difference between the 'flooding' people experience as therapy and what animals have to go through. People are fully informed beforehand and can choose whether or not to participate. Also, they mostly receive one on one counselling from their therapist. Horses are not given a choice, an explanation, or counselling they understand. In addition, often they do not stay in the frightening situation long enough to learn for themselves that there is nothing to be afraid of. Meanwhile their stress level is through the roof and their association with the situation is negative. In my opinion, flooding is not a form of therapy that should be applied to animals. I am aware that many domesticated horses are faced with flooding in all sorts of ways, and sometimes this is entirely unintentional. An example might be taking a horse who has never been outside his paddock and is afraid of various stimuli out to a competition or fair without any practice beforehand.

Luckily, flooding, which may lead to a shut down and learned helplessness on the part of the horse, is applied less and less as a training technique. I also see more and more people searching for training alternatives, both when it comes to riding and general training, in which the horse is not confronted with high levels of stress. I welcome this increased awareness and dialogue, because learned helplessness can be visible and invisible. What, for instance, do we think about a horse who is constantly forced to endure hard kicks with spurs and is impeded by pain in the mouth caused by a sharp bit and rough handling of the reins, thus causing an atmosphere of high tension from which he cannot escape, or the foal that is tied to the pole and has to 'learn' that trying to fight and flee the pole is no use when he is tied up? Which means he stays tied until he gives up.

Learned helplessness is not just passivity, it has a direct effect on the body's functioning. Just like in the case of often activated stress and prolonged stress, it has a negative effect on the cognitive abilities and memory capacity of the horse. Learned helplessness increases the likelihood of a horse developing stereotyped behaviours and depression. It also reduces his motivation to discover new things. There is a serious risk that the horse will get used to pain stimuli, in time causing the threshold at which he responds to pain to rise.[1,2]

STEREOTYPED BEHAVIOUR

Another form of withdrawal, of no longer communicating or responding to stimuli, involves horses who show stereotyped behaviour. As previously mentioned, these are behaviours executed in a repetitive rhythm. Some examples of stereotyped behaviours are weaving, nodding, and cribbing.

The horses I observed showing stereotyped behaviour had been doing it for years. In moments of stress, they would show only one or two calming signals before moving straight to the stereotyped behaviour.

I can imagine how stereotyped behaviour might become such an effective coping mechanism for a horse that he immediately applies it in stressful situations. It is a kind of pacifier that lulls him. I can also imagine that before he learned the stereotyped behaviour, he would have shown possible calming signals or stress signals in this situation.

I have also encountered stereotyped behaviours that were probably rewarded in the past, possibly because the owner subconsciously gave a reaction the horse found pleasant, or by means of a direct reward such as a smile or treat. These stereotyped behaviours were displayed by horses when they were expecting a treat but had not yet received it. This could be a horse who lets his tongue loll out of his mouth, then starts to move his head from side to side so that the tongue flaps back and forth. These are stereotyped behaviours that have been learned and that may also become habits.

DEPRESSION

Unfortunately, some horses are kept in circumstances under which they cannot display their natural behaviour. All forms of unfortunate circumstances occur. Some horses have no contact with other horses. Some horses do not go out to pasture. Some horses have no freedom of choice at all. Some horses have a visible or invisible injury that goes untreated. Some do not receive enough food or water. Some are cold because there is no shelter. Some horses are mentally and physically overtaxed in their training. Some are punished. The list of painful circumstances is long and horses, in particular, literally suffer in silence. The posture I have described that occurs during a 'shut down' can then be held much longer. As an observer, I can only describe it as depressed. It is important to realise that domesticated horses live in a controlled environment. As riders and handlers, we can influence this world. We can choose a stable that allows the horse social contacts, where he can go to a paddock, and where he gets sufficient food and water. We can design his training in such a way that he does not experience pain. We can give the horse freedom of choice and play games with him, all to give him joy in life and avoid depression. The brain has plasticity. Withdrawal, learned helplessness, and depression do not have to be the status quo. Something can be done. The tips in Chapter 5 will provide you with some ways to do this.

If your horse goes into a shut-down mode in response to a stimulus, there are several ways for him to come out of it. It may be that the stimulus that caused it disappears on its own. It may also be that the horse gets used to the new situation in time, after which he can deal with it.

It is also possible that the horse has an astute handler who takes him out of the situation. If this handler then also helps the horse to get used to the disturbing stimulus, makes the horse more independent, and gives him more freedom to choose, then that, of course, is optimal. In this case the horse will no longer have to shut down, because he can handle the situation on his own. This is described in diagrammatic form in the communication ladder below.

4.4 COMMUNICATION LADDER: WITHDRAWAL

Ladder 4.2

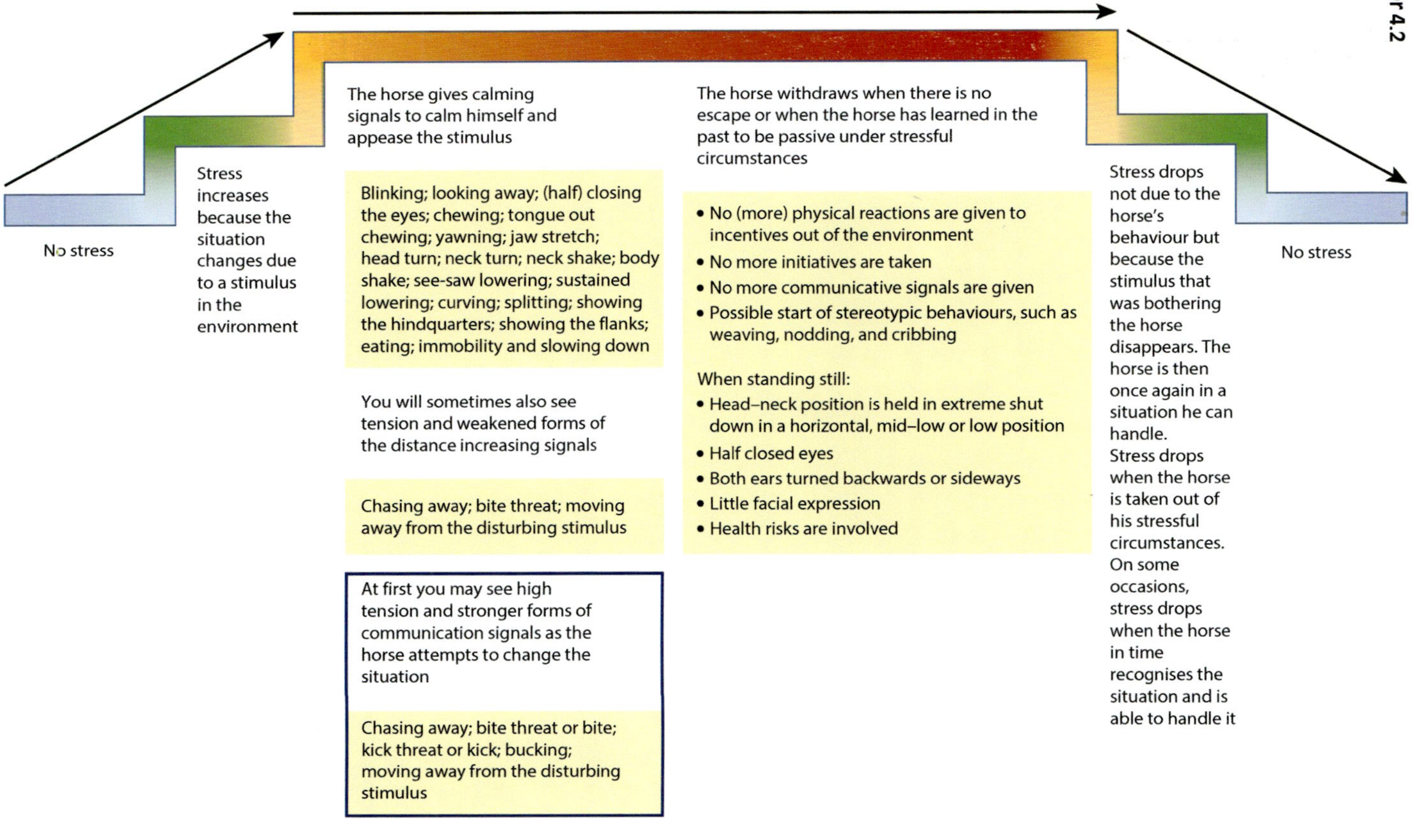

4.5 SUMMARY: NO COMMUNICATION

- There are many reasons why horses may be uncommunicative.
- It may be because they are not interested in a possible back and forth with the other object or the other type of stimulus. It may also be that they do not need to communicate because they can handle the situation without it. Also, new, learned habits may have replaced natural expressions of communication or the horse may be hindered in showing communication signals.
- In response to a stimulus from the environment, the horse may shut down and withdraw (**Fig. 4.1**). A horse who has difficulties with an external stimulus may also show stereotyped behaviour.

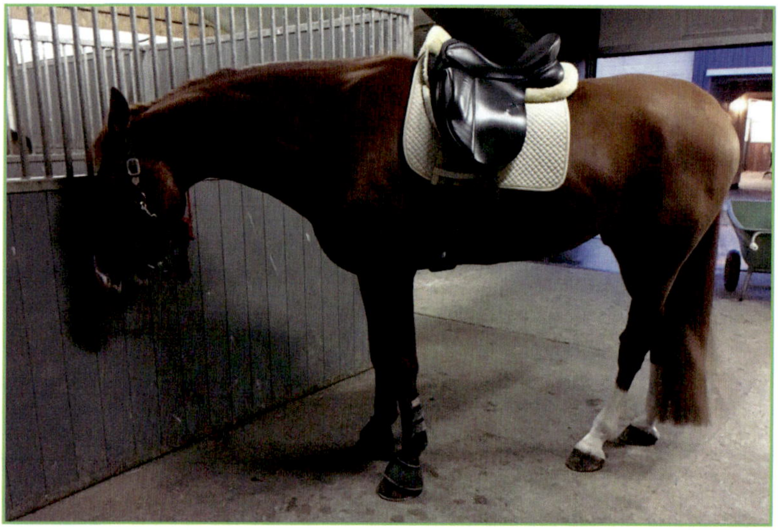

Fig. 4.1 A horse showing withdrawal.

4.6 REFERENCES

1 McGreevy P, McLean A (2010) *Equitation Science*. Wiley-Blackwell, Ames, pp. 99–103.
2 Nyberg J (2014) *The Adaptable Brain*. Lecture at The Dog Symposium, Oslo.

5 *Application of calming signals: how do we help the horse?*

THE TIPS I give in this chapter are aimed at the use of calming signals and knowledge of the variety of signals described in this book. They are intended for riders and handlers who want to better understand, guide, socialise, and train their horse. The tips are useful for anyone who deals with horses, but if you are in a situation that causes discomfort, pain, or fear in you or your horse, or that may cause injury to either of you, the first course of action is to stop and always to consult a behaviour expert and a veterinarian (to rule out physical problems). My tips cannot substitute for this, but they can form an underlying basis and methodology for you and your horse.

THE IDEAL SITUATION

Many horse lovers describe their ideal relationship with their horse as follows: 'I want to be able to communicate without difficulty, so that I understand my horse and he understands me, and for him to do what I ask him to do without problems'. This wish carries an important element, namely the person as the requesting (or demanding) party and the horse as the performing subordinate. Wondering how many rights and desires a horse should be allowed to have in relation to his handler may seem like a philosophical question, but it is much more than that. Considering and formulating what the wishes and rights of your horse are has a clear practical use, and it has an immediate effect on the wellbeing of your horse. It affects his everyday contact with you and others, his ability to learn, and his mental and physical health. What does your horse need? What do you want him to have? Is your horse getting enough food and water? Is your horse cold or too warm? Is your horse in contact with other horses? Does he go to pasture with other horses? Does your horse have enough time to rest, and does he relax when he rests? Is the horse able to do what you are asking him to do, both emotionally and physically? Does he have enough opportunities to make his own choices? The more a horse's needs are met, the better his physical and emotional health will be.

5.1 THE COMMUNICATION LADDER AS AN ASSESSMENT TOOL

When you are responsible for a horse, I believe you have to make sure that he is healthy, not hungry or thirsty, that he has a place to find shelter, that he can go out to pasture for at least a couple of hours a day, and that he is in contact with other horses who make a good match for him. He should be allowed to make choices in order to keep his autonomy and self-determination. From a training perspective, I believe it is necessary for a horse to be guided in such a way that he does not experience any kind of pain. He should also understand and not fear the world people have put him in, and he should be able to handle external stimuli, also without human aide. This is my goal for every horse, regardless of his mental and physical health or level of training, from the Shetlander in the backyard to the Grand Prix horse at the Olympics.

A horse whose needs are met, who has a good relationship with his handler, who is physically and mentally up to the job he is being asked to do, will be cooperative. He is attentive and curious. If you hear yourself saying, 'He (the horse) is just being stubborn', or 'He is angry', your horse has a problem at that point. He is being stigmatised and often receives no more help. After all, you leave someone who is angry or stubborn to 'stew in his own juice' (or worse: you punish him for his negative attitude). It is a status quo in which the horse is the problem and not you. I think this is a missed opportunity. A horse who is described as angry or stubborn is experiencing rising tension. The signals I have been describing apply to him perfectly. Every horse deserves to be able to handle his life and the demands made of him by his handler. That is why it is important for you, as his rider and handler, to know your horse's particular facial expressions and behaviour. Look at the communication ladders and the behaviours that are detailed there. Make a note of which behaviours apply to your horse under what circumstances. Sometimes this requires taking a step back and looking at your horse with fresh eyes. It can happen that riders no longer recognise their horse's tense facial expressions for what they are because they have become so used to their expressions and behaviour. A good way to practise and compare is to watch other horses while they are relaxed at pasture. That expression is the one you want to see on your own horse's face.

You are much better at guiding your horse well when you see when his tension is rising and falling, and when you understand which stimuli are causing it. Immerse yourself in your horse's character. Find out what his goals are, what his motivation is, what is important to him, what he likes and dislikes, and what he likes to eat and not does like to eat. This will allow you to take these matters into account in your cooperation with your horse.

It is very useful to film your horse. A remark heard often from people who sent in video footage for this study was: 'So I sent in the video, but nothing really happened'. However, when those people looked at their own footage again on the computer, they saw many more signals than they had spotted while filming.

This was not just because I pointed these signals out to them, but because they were no longer involved in the situation and in the filming, this gave them the break needed for much better observation.

When does observation become especially challenging? When the horse experiences rapidly changing motivations and emotions and the tension levels that go with them. This creates a pendular representation on the communication ladder. You might see this when your horse is being stimulated by multiple factors in the environment that happen simultaneously or consecutively. Here is an example:

A horse is tied up in the grooming area. Close by is a bucket full of grooming tools, ready to be used. The handler is standing next to the horse. Then, a number of horses are brought out one by one. They pass the horse and his handler in the grooming area. A girl and her Tinker pass by. The horse who is tied up shows a number of calming signals. The Tinker passes. The tied-up horse takes a step in the Tinker's direction but is stopped by the rope. He shows displacement behaviour and then some calming signals. Then a boy and a Shetlander pass by. The tied-up horse shows calming signals. He takes a few steps in the Shetlander's direction, is stopped by the rope, takes a step sideways, and, in so doing, knocks over the bucket of grooming supplies. He shows stress signals, etc.

Your horse may also show a range of body signals if he is placed in an environment that is new to him, causing him to experience shifting tension levels. An example may be a horse who is put in what to him is a new paddock, stall, or grooming area. To your eyes there may be no demonstrable additional stimuli, such as a broom falling over or screaming children (although these may also be present), but in this example it is the new environment itself, in its motionless, 'neutral' condition, that is causing the horse's tension and fluctuating internal state.

Horses who show ambivalent behaviour may also produce a pendular representation on the communication ladder. Ambivalent behaviour occurs when two different behaviour systems are active simultaneously in a horse. Each behaviour system has its own goal and its own strength of motivation. The behaviours from these two systems occurs simultaneously or alternately. For example, a horse may feel light tension as he approaches an unknown object with the goal of learning about it. He may then jump aside with the goal of fleeing and experience high tension. Then he may recover and possibly approach the object again, and so on. Another example:

Vosje has been put out to pasture with three other horses. He has not eaten for a couple of hours and starts to graze with the other horses straight away. Then Lorain, one of the three horses, is removed from the paddock. Vosje stands by the fence gate through which she was led out and whinnies after her. He has light and medium tension features. After 10 seconds, he walks away from the fence and starts to graze again. The tension drops. His motivation is to eat and possibly also to calm himself. After a little while he walks back to the fence and, showing light tension, starts whinnying again.

In this scenario, Vosje has two goals: to be with Lorain and to eat. These alternate, just like their associated tension features. From this position, the tension can develop in two ways. Lorain could stay away too long, Vosje might not be able to handle this, and the tension may continue to increase. In that case he will come to experience high stress and show associated stress signals. It could also be that the tension drops and Vosje just keeps eating and is relaxed. It is also possible that the shifting motivations and emotions remain in the form of alternating waves of tension and relaxation until Lorain comes back. This would produce a pendular representation on the communication ladder in which calm and tension may alternate in different gradations.

5.2 PLANNING AND MANAGEMENT

In the brain, every new learning stimulus is saved together with an associated feeling.[1] A one on one connection is made. If the learning stimulus is perceived to be positive, it will be associated with a positive feeling. A negative learning stimulus is paired with a negative feeling. Naturally, you will want to create a learning environment for your horse in which he saves positive emotional associations. This makes the horse feel more confident about you, his training programme, and the environment in which he lives. It gives the horse a sense of wellbeing and makes him want to cooperate and follow along in your thinking.

It takes planning and organisation to create a positive learning environment. You will want to make a plan that is fully thought through, in which you figure out beforehand which stimuli you might be dealing with. This will allow you to assess if they suit the mental and physical development of your horse. It is also good to try to think of things you may not be able to plan for or manage and consider their consequences. In this case, you should consider if you would want to come up with a new plan or implement a possible stopgap measure.

Knowing what your horse can and cannot handle is the guideline for designing your plan. Reading your horse's body language is indispensable and necessary for doing this. Set regimens are impossible. They do not do justice to the immense variation you see when you work with people and animals. I do, however, follow the guidelines below in my work:

1. Check the horse's health.
2. Create a home environment that suits the character and needs of the horse.
3. Avoid negative experiences.
4. Make a plan to empower the horse so that he can confidently and independently handle stimuli in his environment.
5. Make a plan to teach the horse how to handle certain stimuli or situations he finds difficult and with which the owner or rider has asked for help (assuming these are realistic goals that suit the horse's ability).

LOOKING AT EMOTION, NOT AT BEHAVIOUR

While riding, people often focus on their horse's behaviour or the desired body movements instead of on his emotional wellbeing. This is not because they do not find this aspect important but, so it seems, because they are not used to doing so.

This focus on forcing the horse to perform a desired physical behaviour also happens when a horse is unable to follow a rider's instructions to satisfaction and becomes tense. Often in this situation the rider will sooner reach for a tool to physically force the horse to comply than analyse the situation and take a step back from the task in question so that the tension can ease or disappear. As an example, you might imagine that a horse who is very tense in the arena, jogs and shows flight intentions. To control his behaviour his noseband is tightened, his bit is replaced with a sharper one, draw reins are put on him, force is used, he is whipped, and whatever else people can think of is done to him. These are ways to keep a tense horse under control. They are quick fixes that have bad consequences. Immediately, the horse stays tense and associates this tension with the situation he is in, especially if painful stimuli are also involved. Frequent negative experiences and instances of suppressed tension have a negative effect on his socialisation process, his faith in his rider or handler, his ability to learn, and his health. In the short term this happens because the horse may show distance increasing signals or actually fight or flee, which risks punishment, injury, and the possibility of getting caught in a vicious circle. In time, other health problems associated with chronic stress, as already mentioned in Chapter 3, may surface.

The horse who uses perfect obedience as a coping mechanism to get out of a tense learning situation is just as susceptible to these health risks. These horses are so obedient and are kept so obedient that they also run the risk of becoming so dependent on their rider that they fall prey to learned helplessness. They can no longer stand on their own feet. Saying your horse needs a leader and wants to follow you is not an argument for making him dependent on you or keeping him that way. A leader may also choose to give the people or animals under his charge freedom and opportunities to choose. Compare this with raising children. As they grow older, you give them more freedom and responsibilities. After all, you want to prepare them for an independent life in which you are not there to help. This can happen gradually. At first, they hold your hand as you go through the supermarket, then they place the items on the conveyor belt, then you let them hand over the money, and finally you let them go in and buy something as you wait outside. After that, they can go shopping on their own. If we treated our children as we treat our horses, we would have to hand walk them everywhere, regardless of their age, and we could never allow them to show initiative, let alone decide or do something on their own, not even when they are adults, because this would mean they were disobedient and would have to be punished.

Teaching your horse to deal with life on his own does not imply that your responsibility goes away. Just as with children, you create a framework within which your horse can learn and operate independently. When your child steps into a playground, you take a quick look around and note the see-saws, jungle gyms, and swing seats where he needs to take extra care. You tell him what he can and cannot do, and within that framework he can operate autonomously, make choices, and live his life. The same is also possible for horses. In section 5.10, you will read about all the advantages this brings, and I will give you some ideas.

5.3 CREATING RELAXATION OPPORTUNITIES

So, should a horse never experience any tension at all? No, of course he should. Tension is a part of life and it is unavoidable when you are exploring and seeing, smelling, feeling, learning, and experiencing new things. New stimuli also mean essential mental health and stimulation. It causes new cell production in the brain and promotes neural plasticity.

The key is to find a balance within the tension. You want your horse to be attentive (very low tension) but you do not want him to become stressed (higher tension), in which case the stress replaces the attentiveness. You also want to find a balance between tension and relaxation.

This requires you to take three steps: you need to notice, analyse, and, if necessary, adjust the situation. You will want to avoid continuously higher stress levels and get your horse into a relaxed mode complemented by new stimuli, challenges, and incidental moments of tension. These tense moments will then be such that the horse quickly recovers from them on his own. The tips described below will help you facilitate a relaxed state for your horse and help him maintain this state.

EVALUATE THE EXERCISES WITH A CRITICAL EYE

Ask yourself if the exercises you want your horse to do are realistic, if he can mentally and physically handle them, if he can understand them, and if they are useful. This is especially relevant if the horse has trouble executing the exercises you are asking him to do or is unable to execute them at all. In that case it would be better to abandon the exercise or, if necessary, replace it with something comparable that is more easily accomplished. You can also try the exercise in a different form or apply a more gradual learning process to it.

ALLOW EXERCISES TO TAKE ROOT

Energy, a clear goal, ambition: this might cause you, the rider, to teach your horse something new every time you ride him. This is taxing for the horse, not just physically but mentally, especially if you work or ride him every day. I am a big advocate of having a horse do the same familiar programme three times before I add something new. By repeating the newly learned element three times and thus having the horse recognise it, you give the long-term memory the best chance of saving what has been learned. Also, I want my horse to be relaxed in his work, to feel that he can understand and handle what I ask of him, and to have a pleasant collaboration with his rider. Before he becomes bored with the work, I add a new element. If you are having trouble finding relaxation for yourself or your horse during exercises, or if the horse does not recover during the cool down after riding, make the exercises easier or shorter, or stop the exercise and analyse why you are having trouble with that particular one.

INTRODUCE ONE NEW ELEMENT AT A TIME

'If you introduce a new element, make sure that this is only one new element at a time.'

This tip comes from Anne Lill Kvam, who taught me during her seminars and Nosework Education instruction weekends in scent training for dogs that I attended. The tip has always served me very well with both horses and dogs. It always makes me critically assess my exercises and not combine them or pile them on top of each other because 'it is going so well', causing me to overtax my horse.

HAVE AN ESCAPE PLAN

Coming up with new stimuli and experiences for your horse is fun and necessary. However, try to make your plan as airtight as possible so that you can avoid any possible negative associations your horse may end up having with you or your chosen learning environment. It may mean asking children to talk at a short distance from the horse so that he can have a look at them at his leisure and is not caught off guard. It may mean putting up tape in the stable passageway so that visitors have to keep a greater distance when they walk past your horse's stall.

If, for example, you are planning to take a new route through the forest on your ride, cycle that route once first. Think about what you might encounter on the route and consider if your horse can handle this. If it is impossible to predict how your plan will turn out with one hundred percent certainty, then make another plan where this is possible, or have a plan B ready. This may mean that you do not take rides in the country on Sundays, the day when there are a lot of cyclists and people who let their dogs off the leash out and about. This may mean knowing when the local authorities pick up the rubbish so that you can either steer your horse clear or purposefully approach. Is your horse afraid of cars? If so, do not take him onto a narrow country road where there is no room to get far enough out of the way if a car should pass. Do, however, find a path that allows your horse to watch cars from a safe distance, so that he does not build up tension but forms a positive association with the cars.

If you are taking your horse outside for the first time, make sure you are with a group of well-socialised horses your horse feels safe around and riders who do not mind complying when you want to slow to a walk for a while to allow your horse to emotionally and physically recover. Make sure, for example, that you know of alternative routes when riding in the woods so that you can break off a route and make it smaller.

THE HORSE DETERMINES THE INITIATIVE AND TEMPO WHEN DISCOVERING A NEW STIMULUS

For example, if I have placed a rubbish bag filled with all sorts of interesting scents in the corner of a large paddock, I let my horse determine how and at what speed he wants to deal with the stimulus. Light and medium tension is all right, as long as you think the horse will recover from it in the same session. If, however, I have made an error in judgement and am seeing high tension features or behaviours, then I will place the rubbish bag in a location where the horse is relaxed, but where he can place himself at a greater distance from it, or I will place the bag in a different or smaller form. Next, I will gradually vary the stimulus in order to accustom the horse to the original stimulus. If the horse feels light or medium tension and I think he will relax, then I will let him choose how to deal with the new stimulus. He does not have to approach it. If he chooses to turn around or increase the distance, then that is fine. If the horse takes a break to have a good look at the stimulus, I wait, for however long it takes, without pressuring the horse. This is his decision. I am just an observer; I stay out of it. I will not interfere with his process of investigating and learning. My gift to him is time and relaxation. His gift is the excretion of dopamine, which gives him a powerful feeling of wellbeing.[2] Maybe your horse does not start to investigate the object you put down straight away. Your horse may choose to keep his distance from the rubbish bag, when you had hoped that he would want to rummage through it. But that is the horse's coping strategy at that moment. You will want to support him in it and not force him in any way. When he is more accustomed to objects, his coping strategy will also change. In a healthy horse, curiosity always wins. In my experience, the less you force, the braver your horse becomes in time. You do not want your horse to become overtaxed; you want him to start to see the fun in discovering new stimuli. If this happens, you will see that he no longer looks at new objects with fear or suspicion, but is enthusiastic about approaching and investigating them.

ALTERNATING DAYS OF EFFORT WITH DAYS OF RELAXATION

After a horse has had a day in which he has experienced more tension than normal, I give him recovery days to prevent him from possibly accumulating tension. In this way I prevent moments of incidental stress from becoming chronically raised stress levels. I do undertake useful activities during relaxation days, but only ones I am certain will not cause stress. What that is can differ depending on the horse. My horse, for example, really likes going for a walk and eating along the way. So that is what I do, or I will go tracking with him (see section 5.10). If your horse has handled a difficult situation very well, it is a good idea to follow it up with a relaxation day. That way, the association with the difficult situation that turned out well will have enough time to be properly saved in the brain. If a horse experiences something negative after this positive event, then the negative learning association may come to crowd out the earlier positive learning association.

HELP YOUR HORSE

If a horse finds a stimulus too difficult to handle and experiences medium to high tension, I will choose to help him. Always. An example: my horse has moved to another stall. He is fearful. He kicks the door and whinnies when he hears my voice. I immediately go over to him. Now, you might think that you are rewarding his kicking behaviour this way and that it is better not to go to him, but I disagree. An animal who is tense should receive support. The behaviour of kicking is not what you should look at; you should look at the underlying emotion. That is what you have to respond to. In this example, the horse is kicking the door to attract attention. He is scared and needs support. I give him that support by standing in his stall with him. He relaxes and starts to eat. The more often I comfort my horse, the faster he will relax each time, because his need is being met. Once he relaxes, he stops kicking the door. Imagine that I had not gone over to him, or yelled at him to stop kicking, then my horse's tension would have increased even more. This is counterproductive because I want to get him into relaxation mode as quickly as possible. The same applies to doing obedience exercises when the horse is tense. For example, when the horse is tense and anxiously walking back and forth, making him stand still, of all things, can greatly increase his tension. In that situation it is better to find a compromise and see how you can help your horse lower his tension, but within your chosen framework. You could, for example, hand walk him for a while. This approach is supported by research showing that an animal, or a person for that matter, who receives help in a scary, stressful, or depressing situation is better able to handle that situation.[2,3] This is because the support the horse receives causes the secretion of, among others, the hormone oxytocin, which regulates the amygdala, the fear centre.[4] Oxytocin is seen as the messenger of affection, trust, and connectedness is the brain.[4]

DO NOT PUNISH

Punishing damages your horse physically and mentally. It damages the faith your horse has in you. It causes the horse to form negative associations with an already difficult situation. It makes the horse very tense, which produces a bad learning environment. Punishing is an admission of weakness. When you challenge yourself to no longer punish, you will become a better trainer, because without the punishment methodology, you really have to think, consider what the horse finds difficult, and decide how you are going to solve this by means of good planning. If you need physical punishment in a certain situation, then the situation has not been well thought out or suited to the horse in the first place. If, for example, a horse runs out of the stable and the only way to stop him is to strike him with a whip, then he is already in a situation he is unable to handle. What is the underlying problem? Maybe this horse is afraid of being in the stable. Maybe he has not been trained to be in there alone away from his fellow horses. These potential causes of his behaviour need to be examined and dealt with, not just his running out of the stable. Look at the underlying cause, not just the behaviour. A horse who paces by the fence might be bored or he might have trouble with the location of the paddock. He may calm down if he is moved closer to other horses or if he is brought back to the stable first, or together with a buddy.

GIVING THE HORSE SOME FREEDOM

This allows the horse to act on some of his own motivations, which helps him to stay relaxed. This implies, for example, that you allow your horse to have a look at his surroundings, to stand still for a moment, turn his head, or possibly turn his whole body. While riding it implies allowing your horse to, for example, stretch his neck or look away, enabling him to give a calming signal in order to calm himself or another. It means letting your horse turn away when you are grooming him, for example, allowing him to direct his hindquarters towards an approaching horse or an object that scares him as a calming signal. When you are unloading your horse from a trailer, it implies taking his visual limitations into account and letting him, for example, turn or lower his head so that he can see where he is going. The same applies to riding in the woods. Give your horse the freedom to lower and raise his head so that he can make out his surroundings. If you are afraid to do this and need extra equipment to control him, a ride in the woods might still be too difficult for the both of you, and you should look for an exercise that you can both handle in a relaxed state.

YOU MUST COMMUNICATE

A slap if the horse does not stand still, a yell if he presses his ears back, a jerk on his head if he turns his head away: punishing a horse for communicating or hindering his communication creates tension in the horse, as well as a negative learning environment, and harms his wellbeing, even if, after the punishment, the horse obediently stands perfectly still. By punishing the horse or hindering him, you take away his ability to express himself. In addition, you deprive yourself of the opportunity to find out why he is giving signals or to re-examine your own rules and methods. Communication is a must, as is listening and helping one another.

If your horse is in a stall that is part of a row of stalls, one next to the other, and he has a problem with being fed last, possibly communicating this by pressing his ears back during feeding time and swinging his head with his teeth showing, then I will choose to recognise his feelings and signals and feed him first, even before he starts to show these signals. In my experience, his tension will then no longer be activated, or only briefly and not to a high level, and in time the horse will get a more positive association with feeding time. This is a fundamentally different approach to the method in which you do not feed the horse until he shows the desired passive, signal-free behaviour. This strategy leads to the horse being hungry for longer, his tension rising, and a negative association with feeding time being maintained. Also, a horse who is highly stressed because he is not fed quickly enough will take much longer to figure out that he needs to show passive behaviour in order to get his food. This kind of purposeful reasoning is made much more difficult by the stress he feels. After all, stress reduces cognitive ability. In this example, as well as in other examples in which riders or handlers to do not respond to their horses' signals, I see the following reactions from horses:

1 The horse gives ever larger and more visible signals and his tension rises.
2 Due to having received punishment, the horse does not give incremental signals (he is holding back), but because his tension does increase, it seems to the rider or handler that he is giving an extreme reaction out of nowhere.
3 The horse no longer communicates and blocks everything out.

None of these three reactions are what I want to see, nor do they fit with my intentions and method. By looking at the horse's signals I want to achieve a better interaction with the horse and enable myself to create a plan that is specifically suited to his capabilities. This often requires taking a step back. Communicating also means listening. It means adapting to the wishes and signals of another. If your horse gives a distance increasing signal, such as threatening to kick, respect this. Stop what you were doing. Respect the boundaries your horse draws. Do not punish him. Do, however, make a note of the circumstances under which your horse is doing this so that you can make a new plan, a plan in which the horse does not develop the same level of tension and so does not need to show distance increasing signals. The more you listen, understand your horse's signals, and anticipate them, the more relaxed your horse will become. With that relaxation as a basis, you further educate your horse. Do not be afraid that your horse will abuse your compliance. I have not seen a situation in which a horse sees his handler's acquiescence as a reward, after which he purposefully gives the signal in order not to have to do something. I have, however, seen certain body signals that a horse was re-taught to give on command, such as lifting a foreleg or lolling his tongue out. Calming signals are communicative expressions. The horse responds to stimuli and communicates. This communication differs according to the stimuli and the situation. I have seen horses who were allowed to communicate more, and who were also listened to more, actually start to communicate more. And in my opinion this is a good thing.

ADJUST THE TEMPO AND CALL BREAKS

In my observations I have noticed that horses relax a lot more when the owner does not feel time pressure. Often the clock is a determining factor for the rider. For example, you have to go grocery shopping and attend a birthday party, so if you get to the stable at three o'clock and saddle your horse quickly, you can just get a ride in. The result is quick, efficient treatment of the horse. He is there as an object, receives a petting, sure, but there is less room for contact, communication, and relaxation. What causes tension in the horse is when his handler or rider is walking around at high speed, purposefully and with muscles tensed. It is better to walk with a gait, gaze, and body that is relaxed and at a slower pace so that your muscles are less tense. It also helps to take little breaks in between actions. When you are saddling your horse, for instance, first calmly place the saddle cloth, then take a 1-minute break, let the horse smell the saddle, calmly put the saddle on his back, take a 1-minute break, put the girth on, etc. This is not just important when you have an inexperienced horse, but it is for an experienced horse as well.

ALLOWING TENSION TO EBB BY EATING AND TRACKING

You can let a horse who is tense eat or track. Both the eating and the act of tracking, trying to find food for example, will lower his tension. It is also a good distraction. If your horse does not want to eat or track when he normally enjoys these things, then there is a possibility that he is ill or that his level of tension is too high. In this situation it would be sensible to see if you can do something about the stimulus that is causing the tension, find some other way to help your horse, or remove him from the situation. For example, you could ask people to move further away from his stall, or put him in a different paddock if he is having trouble with some stimuli in the first one.

ADAPT YOUR PROGRAMME TO YOUR HORSE'S WISHES

Take your horse's wishes into account. Enjoy it when he is having fun. The horse adapts to our wishes, so it is only fair to return the favour, to give and take as in any healthy relationship. For example, when you are hand walking him, you can let him choose where he wants to graze. Or when you are riding in the country, you can let him choose the route, which also means accepting this if it turns out to be a very short ride. You can take him to water if you know he enjoys playing in it, or to places with lots of loose sand where he can roll around. You can offer him scent games or other types of games, if that is what he likes to do. And you can create an enriched environment (see section 5.10), enabling your horse to choose the discoveries he wants to make for himself.

Adapting to your horse's wishes may also mean that, if possible, you no longer do an activity, or you do it differently, if your horse dislikes it or finds it less pleasant. Do not pull his mane, for example, but cut it so that he does not feel pain. Or if he dislikes being groomed, you can skip grooming every once in a while or make it shorter. Note that the fact that your horse always stands still very nicely during grooming does not mean that he enjoys standing still for long periods. It can be learned behaviour if he is always tied up and there are no other options. How do you find out for certain if he likes grooming or if he thinks it is taking too long? Release him into a, to him, familiar arena or paddock. Let him explore the arena at his leisure. When he is finished exploring and starts to stand still in one place, go up to him and start to groom him. Do not tie him up for this, and do not give him any verbal or physical commands to stand still. (I am assuming here that your horse is brave enough to take the initiative.) If your horse enjoys being groomed, he will definitely stay in one place and even turn the areas of his body he wants groomed in your direction. If he does not enjoy it, or if he thinks it is taking too long, he will definitely walk away.

5.4 NOT LEAVING YOUR HORSE ALONE AND USING A HAND SIGNAL

As everyone knows, horses naturally live in groups. For a domesticated horse too, living together with other horses is an essential and natural need. During my research I saw horses who, when interacting with people, had trouble being left alone. This could be when the horse was tied up in the grooming area and the owner walked away once or twice to collect grooming equipment. It can also happen when owners leave their horse alone to go and greet or talk to someone. Horses are often left alone at competitions, in trailers, in boxes, or in paddocks. This is normal for people. For many domesticated horses it is still very difficult. As such, depending on their level of tension, they will show calming signals, displacement behaviour, stress signals, or distance increasing signals, in weakened form or at regular strength.

A little planning can prevent these moments for the horse or at least make them shorter and easier, lessening his tension and enabling him to be more relaxed and make more positive associations with his environment. You can have grooming supplies, saddles, and so forth ready at the grooming area so that you do not have to walk away all the time. You can make sure you are fully dressed and ready before you collect your horse. People you wish to talk to can be asked to come to you, so that you do not have to leave your horse, assuming your horse does not mind other people and being part of the whole group. During the conversation you can connect with your horse by, for example, standing by his shoulder with your side turned to him. Or the person you are talking to can be asked to stand where your horse can see and smell them, which also offers him an interesting stimulus he can handle. If your horse has trouble with people, postpone the conversation until you are done with him, or put him back into the paddock and pick him up again after you have finished the conversation. You can also choose to give your horse something to do while you are talking to someone, such as giving him hay to eat. This will make the wait more pleasant for him.

Arrange matters so that you can always stay with your horse if he is uncomfortable being alone. Have someone else fetch the coffee or tea at competitions, bring sandwiches and drinks from home, or arrange for a replacement if you do have to step away.

This all applies especially to horses who are uncomfortable being alone, whether at home or on unfamiliar turf. Practising this is practically useful, but really it is all about empathy. Even if your horse is capable of being alone, it is not nice to treat him like a suit-case you can just put down somewhere and retrieve when you need it.

USING A HAND SIGNAL

When you walk away from your horse, he does not know what your intentions are and when you are coming back. By planning ahead, I try to arrange my interactions with my horse in such a way that I do not leave him alone. But even then it sometimes happens that I do have to step away from him for a second. To give my horse more security when I am gone, I have introduced and practised with a hand signal. I learned this from Turid Rugaas when attending her International Dog Trainers Education course. Turid teaches it to her students. The signal is applicable to dogs, but it is also very useful with horses.

In my case the signal is opening the hand and then closing it again. It can be anything, however. I find this hand signal useful – after all, I always have my hand right there with me. It is also easy to turn it into a natural, automatic gesture and not use it for anything else.

I use the hand signal to tell the horse that he does not have to follow me and that we will be apart for a moment. I am out of sight for a short amount of time but will be back. I practise this in very small steps. At first, I make the gesture when I do not do anything specific with the horse, but I do stay within his sight. I give the hand signal before I start any physical action. 'You do not have come along this time; I have to take care of something myself'. And that is what I then do. I collect hay, for example, or clean something up. These actions are close to the horse, within his view, but you are not involved with him specifically. It takes time to ingrain this signal in yourself, because there will be times when you are doing something in the stable that the horse cannot participate in, but you have forgotten to use the hand signal to tell him this; for example, when you are sweeping the passageway in the evening when all the horses are in their stalls. Once I have become consistent in using the signal, and I have used it with the horse many times, then I will also start to use it when I am going to be out of sight for a few seconds. The number of seconds that I am out of sight can then be increased. However, the goal is not to teach the horse to be alone for as long as possible. It is my horse-friendly choice not to do that. The goal is to give your horse a communication signal that says, 'I will be right back'. It is not a command to 'stay'. I do not use food rewards when teaching my horse this specific hand signal, because I do not want to create tension over an expectation of food.

5.5 USING CALMING SIGNALS YOURSELF

Can horses recognise the non-verbal body language of people? I think humans and horses are naturally so physically different that they do not automatically understand one another. We do not have clearly visible ears, long necks, or tails we can use to give easily readable signals. We stand on two legs instead of four. Because of the differences in build between people and horses, I think horses often interpret our movements differently to how we would want them to. For example, because our eyes are frontal, in the middle of our face, we mostly face the horse full on to look at him. When we walk towards him, we do so frontally, in a straight line. In my opinion, horses have to learn that this is our natural way and if they have not been properly socialised with people, their first encounter with a new person will result in them shying away from these frontal movements coming towards them instead of reading our friendly intent.

By being around people, horses learn and experience what our intentions are and what human body postures, sounds, and behaviours accompany these intentions. In their lives with humans, horses try out and experience which behaviours have a positive and which have a negative consequence for them and adapt their behaviour accordingly. Observation is a part of that learning process.

One of the questions that particularly interests me is whether people can learn to use the body signals of horses so that they understand us better and the communication between people and horses improves. For the past few years I have been trying to find out if I (and others) can use certain calming signals to improve our communication with the horse and offer him more relaxation and clarity. Personally, I have come to the following conclusions:

1 Yes, I can give certain calming signals to the horse. By using these calming signals, I show the horse that I do not want to be in conflict with him and I am able to reduce his tension. It can also give the horse more confidence in collaborating with me.
2 Yes, there are a number of calming signals that I can give to a stimulus together with my horse. In this case, I either follow my horse's lead or guide him. The use of these calming signals reduces the horse's tension over other stimuli. It also gives him greater confidence in me and in a positive collaboration.
3 The calming signals that are very useful in the ways described above, and on which the first two points are based, are splitting, curving, turning the back and flank, doing a head turn, doing a shoulder turn, and standing still.

NOTE: If you choose to give calming signals to your horse, or with your horse to a stimulus, the main message has to be that you as a human being do not want to be in conflict with your horse or the stimulus in the environment. You want to appease the horse and the stimulus. Your behaviour and follow-up movements to or with the horse always have to be in accordance with that message.

The following sections go into further detail about these signals.

5.6 SPLITTING

As described previously (see section 2.17), the horse splits up two parties when he wants to prevent escalation. He also splits when he wants to protect or monopolise valuable objects, animals, or people.

If you notice or predict your horse's tension increasing because of certain stimuli, you can also act as a splitter and with the same goals. As you are splitting, make sure you:

1. Stand in a strategic position between your horse and the stimulus that is making him tense or that you think will make him tense (**Figs 5.1–5.4**).
2. Stand still with a relaxed body posture and relaxed muscles.
3. Have your back or side turned towards your horse.

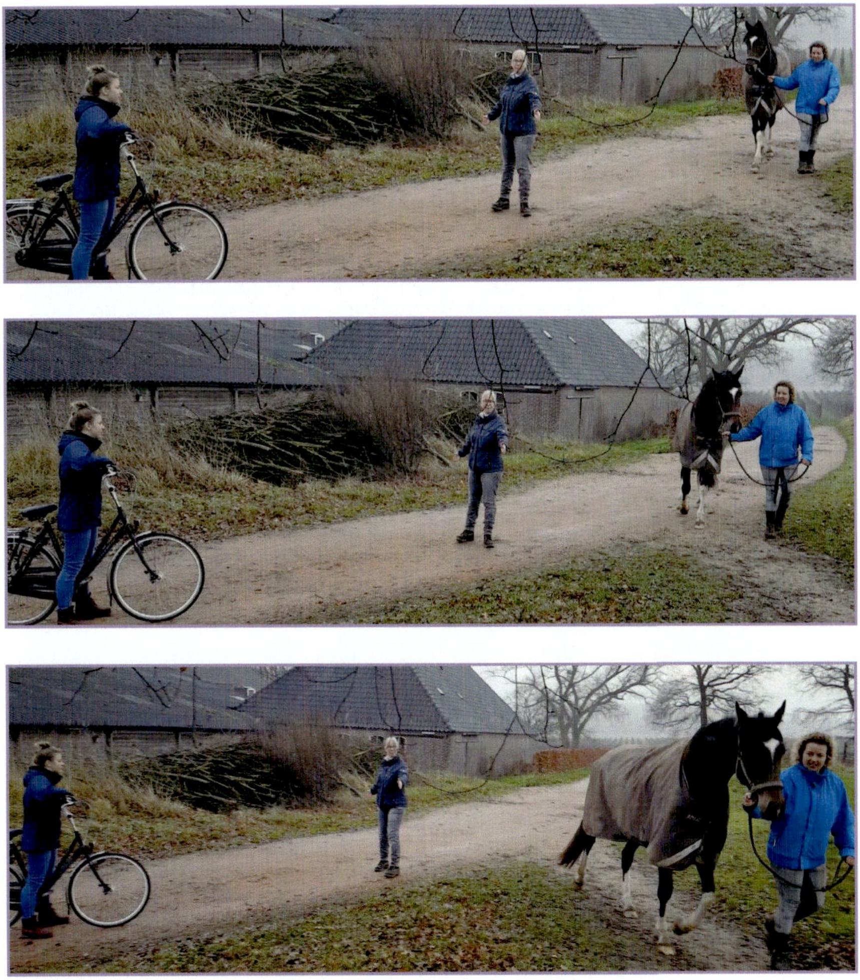

Figs 5.1–5.3 Rachaël splits as a calming signal between Indy and her handler Annemarie and the cyclist, Imke, who is waiting to proceed, straddling her bike.

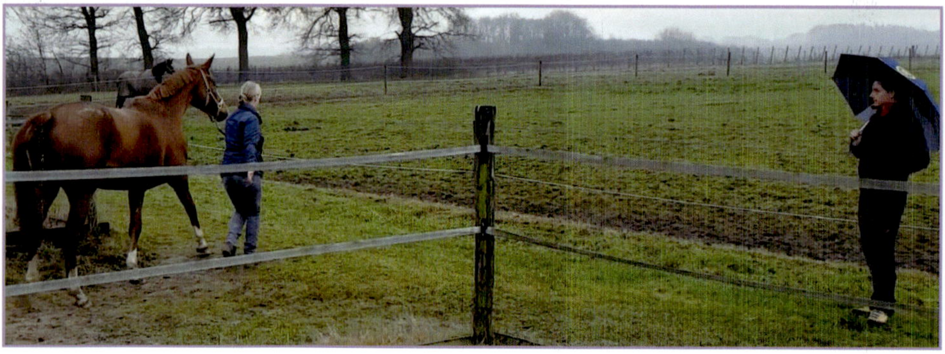

Fig. 5.4 Rachaël splits between Gijs, who stands off to the side, holding an umbrella, and J'adore, giving J'adore a protected position.

If you are hand walking your horse and you are splitting as you walk, then you walk on the side of the horse that has the stimulus. Your horse then walks on the outside. You also turn your upper body frontally towards the possibly disturbing stimulus. However, in a situation where you have the help of an extra splitter and the tension is very light, you might decide not to walk on the side that has the disturbing stimulus. In **Figs 5.1–5.3**, Annemarie is aware of Indy's low tension and does not change her position. If Indy's tension was higher, she would have walked between Indy and the cyclist even with Rachaël at hand to act as splitter.

When you act as a splitter, you give your horse support. You protect him. But this protection does have to be reliable for the horse. If, for example, you are splitting between your horse and two toddlers who are making a noise and you do not pay attention, allowing the toddlers to get near your horse, then you are not a dependable splitter. When you are splitting, the goal is to actually make your horse safe and make sure he is not approached by the stimulus you are splitting him from. It is satisfying to notice when your horse learns that you are a good splitter and he comes to stand behind you in a situation of, in his eyes, possible danger. In this situation you protect him and then continue his socialisation to empower him and make him able to deal with stimulus.

Some examples of situations in which you can split are described below, as well as additional points about splitting:

- When your horse is tied up in the grooming area, you can split when other horses are passing.
- You can split between your horse and, for example, a dog who comes up looking for attention.
- You can split between your horse and certain people or sounds when he is in the stable or at pasture.
- Split when your horse needs it. If your horse is completely comfortable with screaming toddlers, dogs off their leash who want to be friendly, people of all kinds, then you do not have to split and protect your horse. After all,

your horse is perfectly able to handle the situation and can enjoy all the stimuli around him.

- I do not advise splitting up two horses at pasture who you suspect will get into a conflict. Human speed and reaction time is much slower than that of horses. We can use certain signals and horses respond well to them, but that does not mean that we know the entire language of horses and can apply it in possibly highly tension situations. You want to avoid getting hurt. I prefer to spend much more time on a good match between horses and a sound introduction than on damage control.
- If, under extraordinary circumstances, I do split between horses loose at pasture, I will only do so if I know the horses well, can see that their internal motivations and emotions are mild, and am confident that they can see and understand my signal.

5.7 CURVING IN AN ARC

A horse who walks in a curve as he approaches an unfamiliar object, animal, or other stimulus is being careful. He does not want escalation and uses the curve as a calming signal to appease the stimulus and calm himself. He can also use the curve to observe the stimulus in a way he finds comfortable. For people, making an arc in relation to a stimulus is unnatural. Our eyes are at the front of our skull and so we approach stimuli in a straight line. Additionally, we know the world around us and generally do not fear it, so making a curve has no added value to us. When horses are being hand walked or ridden, it is on a 'human' straight line, passing objects, passing people, passing animals. This may cause added tension in horses who have not yet been fully socialised. Riders and handlers can lower this tension in the horse by allowing him to make a curve if he wishes, following along in it if necessary. We can also initiate an arc ourselves. We can do this when we are riding a horse, walking a horse, or want to approach a horse. The horse's level of tension determines the size of the arc. If your horse is very tense, then make a large arc. If your horse is lightly tense, then make a small arc. If your horse is relaxed, you do not need to make an arc at all, or you could just make a very slight curve. Below are some examples of when curving can be useful.

CURVING IN RELATION TO OTHER HORSES OR ANIMALS AT PASTURE

When my horse is at pasture with several other horses and I want to take only him out, I walk him past the others in an arc. In this way, my horse and I are giving the other horses a calming signal. It appeases them and allows my horse to stay (more) relaxed.

CURVING IN RELATION TO 'SCARY' STIMULI

When I am riding on country roads, I want to be very visible. I wear an orange safety jacket and ride near the middle of the road. If I see a stimulus I think my horse will respond to, I make an arc, literally going around the problem (**Figs 5.5–5.8**). By not forcing the horse to approach the object in a straight line or pass very close to it, his tension lessens. Even better for the horse is when you loosen the reins a bit, allowing him to give any calming signals he wants, such as a neck turn or head turn, or a lowering of the head and neck. Making an arc is especially useful if the horse feels light tension. If the horse has no trouble with the object, then of course you can walk past it in a straight line. If the horse has a lot of trouble with the object, make your curve much wider. However, if you do want to use curving, make sure you choose paths that offer sufficient room for wide curves and avoid paths that are too narrow for a while until your horse has been socialised enough that a small arc on a narrow path is sufficient to keep him relaxed.

The curving described above, which you can use as a calming signal while riding, is also applicable to hand walking. However, in this case it is important that when you are leading your horse through a curve by hand, you make sure that you are

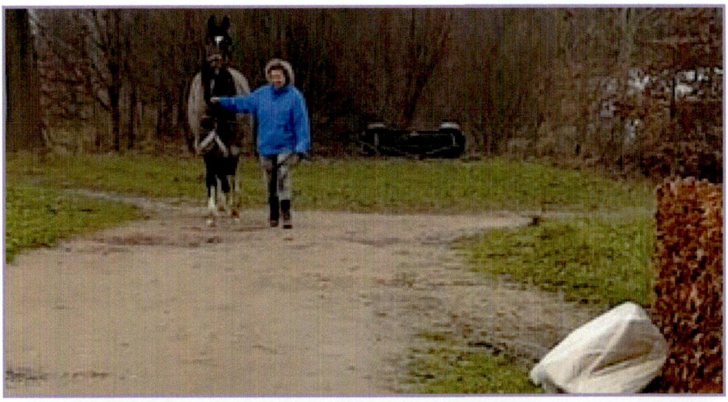

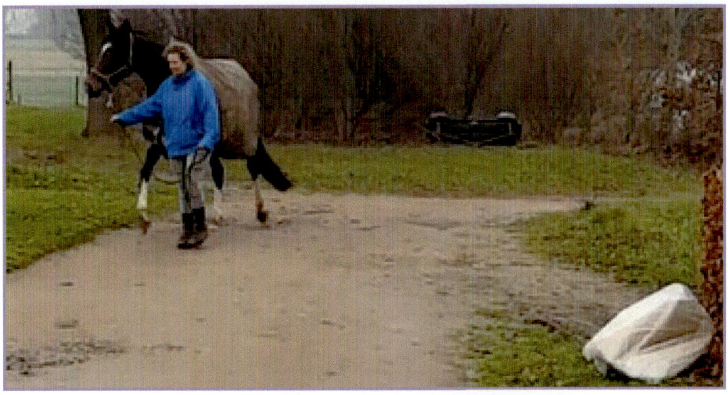

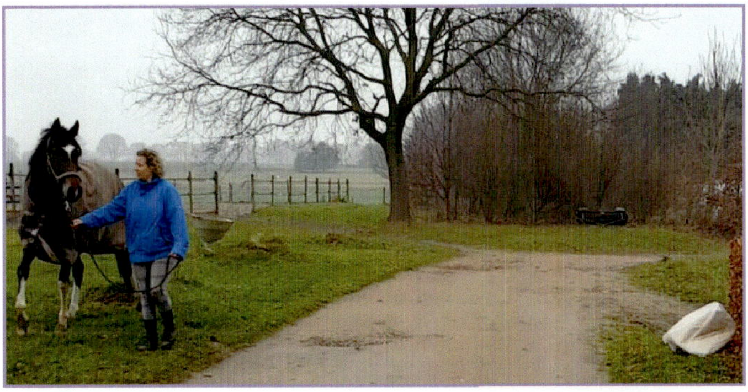

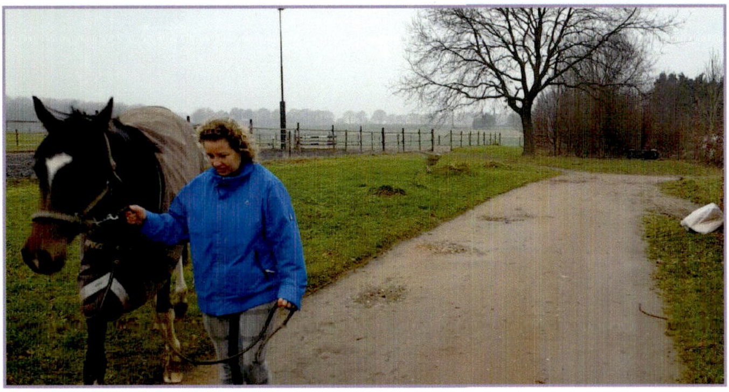

Figs 5.5–5.8 ***Top:*** Annemarie leads Indy down the path. By the hedge on the right there are two plastic bags Indy has not yet seen. ***Upper middle:*** As a calming signal towards Indy, Anne Marie starts a curve. ***Lower middle:*** She continues the curve. ***Bottom:*** She returns to the path.

splitting between the horse and the stimulus to which the two of you want to be polite and which you do not want to provoke. In that way you combine two calming signals: splitting and curving. Also, practically, you make sure that when your horse jumps away from the stimulus, he jumps away from you instead of towards you. This implies that the horse will sometimes walk to your left and sometimes to your right, depending on the situation.

CURVING AS A STRATEGY FOR APPROACHING A FRIGHTENED HORSE (FIGS 5.9–5.12)

When you are approaching a horse who is building up tension because of you or your approach, curving is a very useful tool. The arc you use when approaching a skittish horse can be as large as it needs to be. Focus on an imaginary spot next to or in front of the horse's head or shoulder. When approaching this type of horse, it is very useful to turn your shoulders and navel away from the horse. It is strange to walk this way, but this body posture, just like the arc itself, lessens the horse's tension. When you make the arc, walk calmly with your muscles relaxed. During the curve you can also give other calming signals, such as turning your head or shoulders away in a fluent movement and then back into position. You can also stand still as calming signal when you see the horse give a calming signal. Then you can assess whether that has been enough practice for the day or if you can keep going after a short break. The latter is possible if you think the horse can handle the exercise, will recover from any possible light tension, and can end the exercise on a positive emotional note.

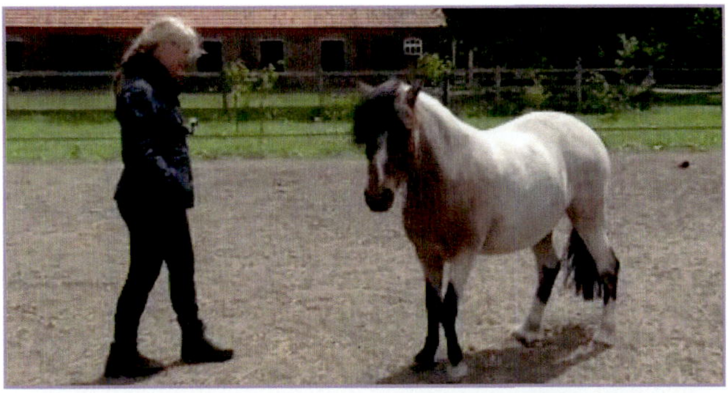

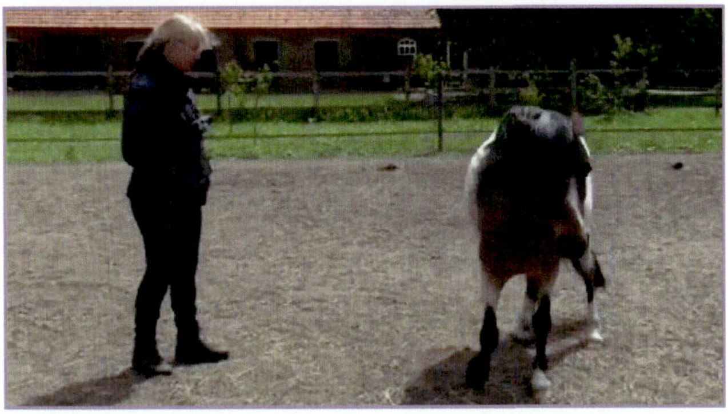

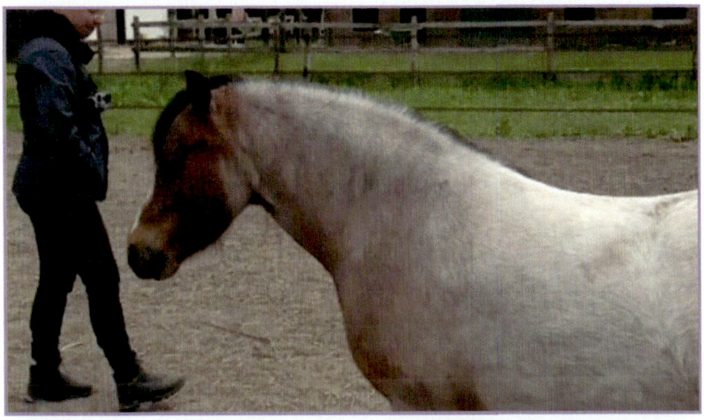

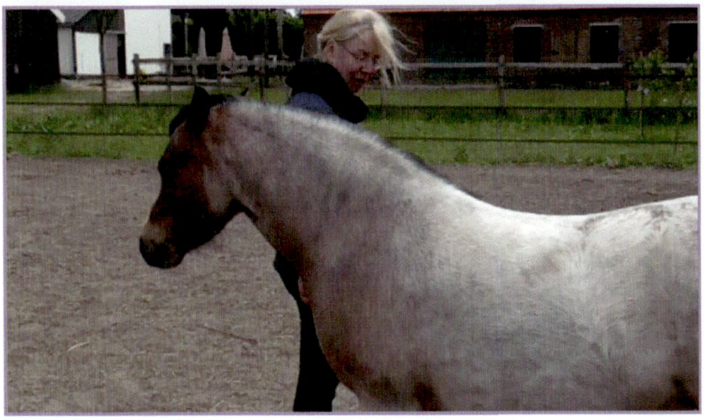

Figs 5.9–5.12 Indy finds it difficult when people other than her owner approach her. Compare the photos. ***Top:*** I approach Indy, walking slowly, but my upper body is turned towards her more frontally. ***Upper middle:*** The moment I turn my navel towards her, she walks away. ***Lower middle:*** I walk towards Indy in a small, slow, relaxed arc. My shoulders are turned a bit to the left. I do not turn my navel towards Indy. ***Bottom***: This allows me to approach Indy and stroke her. During this brief stroking session, lasting only a few seconds, Indy has her eyes open or half closed.

5.8 SHOWING THE FLANK OR BACK

Horses show their flanks and hindquarters to stimuli to indicate that they want to pause the communication or end it altogether. If a horse gives this signal to another horse, then the turning of the flank or hindquarters does not provoke the other horse. The opposite, in fact. The other horse recognises these calming signals and immediately responds in a way that prevents conflict, often by showing his own flank or hindquarters and also starting to graze.

If a horse is turned frontally towards another horse, then he intends to approach that horse (the chest and forelegs indicate the intended direction of movement). As stated before, because of the position of our eyes in our skull, people often stand frontally facing their horse. It seems to me that the horse interprets this stance as an intention by the person to move towards him. This causes anxiety in some horses. I have noticed that in dealing with such horses it helps to turn my side towards them instead of facing them fully. I want to prevent horses who have become so used to people that they no longer show any outward signs of tension despite having an elevated heart rate or raised blood pressure when I face them full on; therefore, I have taught myself the habit of standing with the front of my body and my shoulders turned away from the horse wherever possible. This can be when I am talking to someone in front of a horse's stall or when I am watching a horse at pasture, in which case my body is turned away from him, but I turn my head slightly so that I can still look at him. This can also be when I am putting a halter on a horse or a saddle cloth, or when visitors are standing in front of a horse's stall and I can see that the horse is having trouble with this. In this situation I will ask the visitors to turn their backs or sides towards the horse, which reduces his tension. If the horse remains tense, I will ask the visitors to stand further away from the horse and I will split between them and the horse.

Turning your back or side to the horse is a good tool in any case when it comes to horses who have not yet been fully socialised with people. You can have people stand a way off from the horse with their sides or backs turned towards him. The horse can then take in the sight and scent of the people and feel less provoked because of the calming signal.

However, horses who are very free around people, or perhaps need attention, or are used to being given food after begging for it, might actually become more active when you turn your back on them. They will nibble at you or sniff your pockets to see if they might be able to nudge you into action. Their need for attention or food is higher than their internal need to answer this calming signal.

CHOOSING THE RIGHT POSITION

Allowing your horse to show a stimulus his flank or hindquarters, or positioning him that way yourself, is also a technique you can use to help your horse observe an object that is giving him light tension. You can apply this when you know the horse does not want to approach the object, but you find it necessary to practise with it nonetheless. These can be intermediary steps that you take until the horse wants to approach the object on his own.

What you are doing here is copying the behaviour horses display on their own when observing objects they do not yet trust. In moments like this, when there is light tension, horses will want to appease the object and themselves by turning their hindquarters or flanks towards it and also possibly starting to eat. You copy this and let the horse turn his hindquarters towards the object at some distance from it, then stay there like that for a while. A next step might be turning the horse's flank towards the object. I let him graze during this if there is grass. If not, I put down hay for him to eat. The horse will indicate for how long he wants to do the exercise. If he wants to leave the situation, I always follow him. If the horse is having trouble with the exercise, I increase the distance between him and the object, or I make the object smaller, or I introduce very short practice sessions in which I repeatedly take the horse in and out of the situation so that breaks and short practice sessions alternate.

NOTE: If your horse is not experiencing light tension but is experiencing high tension, for instance because you are too close to the object and you turn his hindquarters towards it, your horse may interpret this turning around as a cue to flee. Therefore, it is important that you recognise the tension features in his face and the signals he is giving. If there is doubt, leave sufficient room between you and the object; better too much than too little at first.

This method is contrary to the method that is most often used: turning the horse's head towards the object that is causing high tension. Often the horse who is feeling high tension will then freeze in response. I see riders using this freeze reaction as a workable temporary solution, for example, when they are riding by the side of a narrow road and a lorry approaches. The riders turn their horses so that they are facing the lorry. Because the horse freezes due to high tension, the riders can wait for the lorry to pass by and then continue their ride. However, with this method the horse forms a negative association with the object he is afraid of. It is one way to deal with a situation, but not a solution to the real problem. I am not a advocate of this method. Also, I would choose to avoid narrow roads if my horse was still so frightened of lorries that he would freeze if one should pass. I would not take roads such as that until I had practised enough so that my horse could handle a confrontation with a moving lorry.

If you have to tie your horse up, for example when the farrier is coming, you can also take your horse's literal position into account. If there are other horses present with whom he is not yet entirely comfortable, he will be better able to relax if he has his hindquarters turned towards them.

Also consider where the hay is put down in the stall. If your horse is housed next to a horse who gives a lot of distance increasing signals to your horse when eating, place your horse's hay in the opposite corner, so that your horse can eat with his hindquarters turned towards the other horse. This lowers the tension in your own horse and perhaps calms the other horse as well. Should the relationship between the two of them improve during feeding time, you can place the hay in such a way that your horse has his flank turned towards the other horse.

5.9 STANDING STILL

When, during a ride or a walk, a horse stops and stands still, there is always a reason for it, even if we cannot discern it. It may be that he does not trust something he sees, hears an unfamiliar sound, or smells something he cannot place. When this happens, I see a difference between horses and people. People appeal to their problem solving ability pretty quickly. The 'problem' of standing still and refusing to walk has to be solved. The horse is spurred on, he is talked to, the rider dismounts, pulls on the horse, or sometimes even kicks or hits him. In these moments we are clearly less patient than the horse, who is taking much more time to figure out what is bothering him and whether he can continue safely. It is too bad that we do not have the patience to give the horse time to stand still, look around, listen, and feel. Not giving him that time makes him tenser and possibly gives him a negative association with his rider or handler and the situation he is in, when the standing still could also be a learning experience. First, it offers you, the rider, a chance to find out which stimulus your horse is having trouble with. You can include this in his practice programme. It also offers you a chance to practise your flexibility and patience, should you be bothered by the fact that your ride is not going as planned. But the biggest advantage, I believe, is that you can work on and practise your horse's own ability to deal with stimuli, because you have landed in a situation in which your horse is standing still because something has alarmed him. I will explain these points further.

Imagine that your horse is standing still because he feels apprehensive about something. Do not try to rush things. Adjust your plans, because the ride is already deviating from how you had planned it. Think of the advantages for the moment. Your horse is disquieted about something. You can practise with him right there and then. What are you going to do? Nothing. Give your horse the time he needs to listen, watch, and smell until he considers it safe and decides to continue. This has a great many educational benefits: you keep his tension from rising, thus preventing him from associating a negative feeling with the stimulus, the location, or you; you do not cause a fight or flight response to be triggered; and you do not put your relationship under pressure. What your horse learns and experiences is that he can take all the time he needs to find out whether an object, person, animal, or situation is safe. This keeps the horse from becoming dependent on you and makes him independent instead. You give the learning process over to the horse. When he decides that the object is safe and it is all right to pass, he will have done this by himself. That is a huge boost to his confidence and it will also have a very positive effect in the future. The horse's self-esteem will grow and he will become braver and braver. The time you have to wait for the horse to decide to proceed when there are scary objects (of course, assuming he is not punished when he does not do it) will become shorter and shorter (particularly if you also do the exercises described in section 5.10). When applying this method I have never waited longer than 25 minutes before the horse has decided to proceed on his own after an initially difficult stimulus. After that, the times rapidly became shorter and shorter, until the horse just kept going when there were difficult stimuli. If you do not like long waits, remember that this method has long-lasting positive results, because the horse is developing life skills that he will further build on in the future.

However, with this method it is important that you know whether your horse has light or high tension. If your horse is staring at an object, frozen as if nailed to the floor, ready to bolt at any second, then this method is not yet an option. Your horse is not ready for it. The only choice you have in this situation is to increase the distance between the horse and the object, which means adjusting your ride, walk, or plan. In practice this will turn out to be increasing the distance to the stimulus, allowing your horse to watch, smell, and hear from a distance until the stimulus possibly goes away on its own and you can continue on your way. If the stimulus does not go away and your horse's tension stays high, you can choose for you and your horse to turn back from the object. This is not a sign of weakness but, in fact, a sign of strength. After all, you want to put your horse in situations he is able to handle so that he becomes emotionally stronger and starts to gain confidence in your leadership and parenting. In this case, however, it is good to remember the stimulus your horse had trouble with and make a plan by which he can get used to it and can function more autonomously. This way, you will be able to pass objects that used to inspire intense fear. If you cannot increase the distance, cannot go back the way you came, and cannot take an alternative route, you may want to hand walk your horse. Some horses respond well to this. You can also have your horse walk at the centre of a group of horses who are not afraid. But these are emergency solutions. Knowing where you will be riding, planning the route, and first cycling it, for instance, are important parts of a horse's socialisation. And although you cannot control all the elements on the road one hundred percent of the time, some occurrences are predictable if you go through a local newspaper first. It will tell you, for example, when the local authorities are going to mow the green areas, when there is a national cycling day, when the rubbish is being picked up, or if the motorcycle club is heading out.

5.10 MAKING YOUR HORSE MORE INDEPENDENT: EMPOWER YOUR HORSE

Designing a programme for a horse that details riding goals is a given for many riders. However, drawing up a structured programme for the horse's emotional development is much less common, and this is when it can do so much good.
A horse who is able to deal with stimuli in our environment independently, without fear or help, has:

- Increased reasoning ability.
- Increased memory capacity. He is better able to remember lines of reasoning.
- Increased motivation to try new things.
- Increased inclination to start and maintain social relationships.
- Increased happiness in life and enthusiasm for activities.
- Decreased fear and aggression responses.
- Decreased overreactions.
- Decreased fear of new things.
- Decreased risk of development of chronically high stress levels, depression, lethargy, and learned helplessness.
- A healthy immune system, with a lower chance of developing ailments that can be stress related.

Brains have plasticity. They can adapt to the ever-changing circumstances of life, even until a very great age. These adaptations and changes occur on several levels. Because of stimulation:

- The number of receptors that send information multiplies.
- The amount of information that passes through the receptors increases.
- Blood circulation in the activated area of the brain improves, causing more cell activity.
- New cell structures are created in which new neurons literally form new pathways along which new information is transported.

This applies to every horse, regardless of his mental health. If a properly thought out programme is applied and changes are made to the way the horse lives and the way he is treated, the horse's brain will change, as will his physical and emotional health This applies to healthy horses, but also to horses suffering from mild or severe depression, learned helplessness, or chronically elevated stress levels.

Making your horse more independent, less reliant on you, more capable of dealing with the world, and happier and more relaxed in life, with all the stimuli that come with it, is a training choice you can make for every horse in every situation. What is needed for this?

GIVE YOUR HORSE CHOICES

Self-determination, the ability to influence your environment, the ability to make choices: it enhances the joy of life of horses and is a direct counter to the aforementioned learned helplessness, passivity, and possible lethargy and depression. It is therefore a good idea to think about self-determination and any choices you are able and willing to let your horse make on his own.

When you give your horse choices, it is important that they are actual choices, not choices that are steered by the owner. Putting a horse in a standard paddock and saying he is free to choose where he goes inside it and which blades of grass to eat is not the type of choice I am talking about. The choices I am referring to must have value to the horse and be real deliberations. For example:

- The horse may take the lead when you are hand walking and choose where the two of you go (**Fig. 5.13**).
- The horse may choose where the two of you go when you are riding outside the arena.
- The horse may choose which paddock he wants to be placed in.
- The horse may choose between carrots and apples (offer one in each hand and see if he has a preference), or make other feeding decisions.
- The horse may decide how long the ride will last.
- The horse may decide when he wants to take a break.
- The horse may decide for how long he wants to be groomed.
- The horse may indicate whether or not he wants to approach a new stimulus. He is not forced to do either.
- The horse may indicate when he wants to take a break during physical therapy or during any treatment being offered.

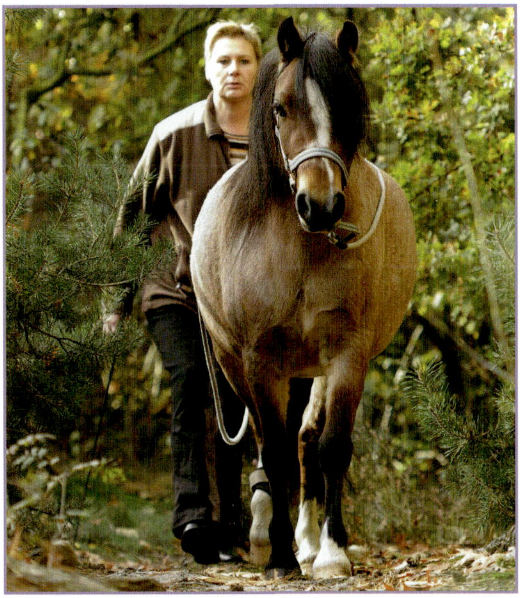

Fig. 5.13 Ristin and Indy are out for a walk. Indy is taking the lead on where to go.

If you know what to look for, the horse will show you what he wants. Here are a few ways in which a horse points:

1 By looking in the direction he wants to go in a high, upright posture. Both ears face forwards. He does not blink. The horse stands still and does not move (the posture is comparable to that of a horse who is trying to figure out a stimulus).
2 The same posture as in 1, except that now the horse repeatedly moves his nose back and forth a couple of centimetres in the direction he wants to go or on which he wants to focus.
3 The same posture as in 1, except the horse now also moves his head and neck. He points his head in the direction he wants to go. He can also possibly take a number of steps in that direction or simply walk over there. If he is hindered in his walk, he may paw.
4 By using his nose to point and actually touching the item that he wants you to pay attention to. For example, if a horse wants food, he will literally go over to his feeding trough and touch it with his nose.

Before a horse starts to point in these different ways, he may first make eye contact with you. If your horse does not feel like doing something you want to do, and he has the freedom to express this, he will show it by giving calming signals and/or turning or walking away from you.

REDUCE YOUR CONTROL AND COMMANDS

When you give your horse more freedom of choice, it is important that you can guarantee his and your safety. Think carefully about the setting in which you give your horse choices and if you always want to integrate this into your lives, or as much as possible, or instead assign certain moments in your horse's life in which he has opportunities to choose. Give your horse choices when you are able to fully gauge the situation and see that the horse can choose safely.

You have to find a balance between the times when you give your horse freedom and the times when you choose and he follows you. If the two of you, and you personally, are doing this for the first time, there may at first be a period in which both of you try to find new boundaries: your own boundaries, but also what you find acceptable for your horse. Some owners prefer to link a clear signal to this. For example, when they have a clear plan in mind and the horse is allowed to make his own choice, owners will say something like, 'All is clear'. They can also give a body signal or a vocal indication like, 'Your turn' when the horse is free to choose and they will follow. If the need arises for them to take back control, they will give another body signal or vocal signal such as 'Done' or 'My turn'. Often, however, it is unnecessary to express who wants what. In time you will find your own mode for it. If your horse knows that he is allowed to move during grooming, he can show you where he wants to be groomed by walking backwards and forwards. You do not need a signal for that. When you are hand walking your horse and letting him lead the way, he will naturally lead you where he wants to go. That way you get to see the places he wants to visit. Is he looking for new stimuli and does he want take new paths or find new objects, or does he play it safe by staying in familiar places?

Examine your own behaviour and analyse how many verbal and non-verbal commands you give. Are all of them really necessary? Can you let go of some of them and give your horse more freedom?

INTEGRATE GAME ELEMENTS INTO YOUR SHARED LIFE

Playing has a very beneficial effect on a horse's wellbeing and on his brain. The opioids and dopamine that are released in the brain during play give him a euphoric feeling. Play also seems to be adequate medicine for depression and appears to be able to repair parts of the brain that have been damaged by stress.[5]

If, on top of all this, you are also able to devise games that cognitively challenge your horse, then you are really doing great work, but this can be a challenge. Figuring out a game is something the horse does only once (possibly spread over multiple tries, if the game is especially challenging). After all, once you have figured out how a magic trick works, you have figured it out once and for all.[6] Say you come up with a game in which you float an apple in a water trough and you invite your horse to see if he would enjoy trying to get the apple out. If he accepts, he will try to grab the apple several times. While doing so, he will discover that he can hold his breath under water and also that he can blow bubbles when his nose is underwater. In this case, the first time he manages to grab the apple, and the first time he finds out about being able to hold his breath and blow bubbles, is the time you mentally stimulated him and appealed to his cognitive ability. Therefore, it is important to realise that the next time you play this game, it does not stimulate anything new in his brain. The discoveries have been made. The apple in the water has become a rote game.

I use three types of play, which I will explain in more detail below:

1 Making and visiting enriched environments.
2 Tracking games.
3 Games that stimulate the senses.

ENRICHED ENVIRONMENTS

You create an enriched environment by temporarily placing new elements in an existing large practice space, thus enriching it. These new elements can be very varied.

For example, blankets that you place on the ground (and of course if the blankets have a special smell it makes it extra stimulating for the horse). You can also think of cardboard boxes in all sizes, a bag full of plastic you have collected, a crate full of empty plastic bottles (without lids), a stick, or an inflatable swimming ring. I usually rummage around in my shed at home and bring some stuff. Ordinary, everyday items from in and around the house are very interesting to examine for a horse:

a chair, a broom lying on the ground, a folding step stool, a jumping rope, a dog leash, a grocery bag, or little flags on a string flapping in the breeze.

An enriched environment stimulates the horse to make choices and to smell, taste, and touch things. It provides new stimuli and mental stimulation and leads to a better understanding of our world and better socialisation. Discovering different things also causes the production of endorphins, which brings about a feeling of wellbeing.

There are several golden rules for a good enriched environment.

The items are safe

The items that are put down must be safe. They should not be too small, leaving no chance for the horse to eat them. It must not be possible for small parts of items, such as bottle caps, to be chewed off larger items. There should be no handles on bags on which the horse's legs can get caught as he walks.

The space is big enough

You place the items in a part of your enriched environment, but a large part of the space remains empty. In that way the horse is not flooded with stimuli and overtaxed, and he can decide the distance from which he wants to observe the items and how he wants to approach them. He can also regularly withdraw if he wants a mental break, before possibly going back to examine the items again. This is why the space in which you place the items needs to be large, such as a paddock, field, or an arena. Imagine that you place your items in a small stall and the horse cannot distance himself from them. Then you are not giving him a choice. You are forcing him to interact with the object and are possibly overtaxing him. This is not what is supposed to happen.

Start small, easily, and calmly

If your horse is careful in approaching things, make sure the environment is calm and quiet when your horse is examining the items. If, when the horse is smelling a plastic ball for the first time, a child suddenly makes a loud noise, the horse may be startled by the noise and associate this shock with the object he is examining or the entire setting. Also, in the beginning, do not drag items around. This may in fact increase the fear. Regardless of the horse, you want to start and end in calm relaxation. To achieve this, it is better to have an enriched environment that is too easy than one that is too difficult. You can change an enriched environment each time.

The horse decides the pace of discovery: the handler does not force anything

You can build an enriched environment and release your horse inside it. You can also choose to hold your horse on a long rope and follow him. Obviously your horse should be used to this and not respond to it with tension.

The goal of an enriched environment is to make the horse more independent, so that he comes to see how much fun it is to discover new stimuli. This is why it is crucial not to force a horse to interact with the object; pull the horse towards it, lure him over with treats, call him over, or jump over objects yourself to demonstrate how much fun it is. The underlying emotion in case of force is not positive. If you are forced to get over your fears, your sense of fear increases and you are less inclined to discover new things. If you lure him with food, your horse comes over for the food, not to discover the item. If you talk and walk around a lot, you distract the horse from his own discoveries. The same is true if you turn the enriched environment into a touching exercise, in which the horse is rewarded for touching things. Do not do this. It turns the whole event into an obedience exercise, and you are not giving your horse a chance to develop on his own.

Horses who have lived very controlled lives and who are literally not allowed to put a foot wrong by their owners often do better at discovering items when their owners are far away or not present at all. I see the same thing with scent games. If I throw some treats on the ground when the owner is not there, the horse will search for them and eat them. If the owner is present, some horses will, under the same circumstances and using the same food, no longer take the initiative. This is not only because they might have learned that their owner does not allow them to show initiative, but perhaps also because they associate food with their owner. The owner is then a type of slot machine that ejects a food reward. In this case, searching for food themselves with the owner present can be difficult at first for some horses.

If this is the case for your horse, ask someone else who the horse is comfortable with to mind him. Stay at a smaller distance yourself. When your horse is enthusiastically searching, reduce the distance towards him in steps until you can stay close, while he is not distracted by you. This can happen in one session, or it may take multiple sessions. I have experienced that the fun of discovery will win out over eventual obedience!

Use your knowledge of language signs

Look at your horse and study the calming signals or other language signs he may be using. See if your horse is building up tension or not. Watch to see which objects cause tension and which do not. If your horse only shows calming signals when he has light to medium tension, you can give him some time. He can stand at a distance and watch. That too is learning.

If you see features of higher tension, possibly in combination with distance increasing signals, then you have unintentionally made the enriched environment too difficult after all. If this is the case, you can lead your horse away, allow him to calm down, change the enriched environment, and let him try again. If your horse is relaxed but still does not approach the objects, you yourself can walk in amongst the objects very slowly. You should walk alone when you do this, not holding your horse. You can also, in an exception to my earlier advice not to lure the horse with treats, place food on top of the objects. However, I only do this once or twice. After that, the fascination over discovering new items takes over from the food.

An enriched environment does not always have be specially built (**Fig. 5.14**). Sometimes it just presents itself. If you have an eye for it, you can give your horse a real-life enriched environment (**Figs 5.15, 5.16**). When riding in the country, for example, you can stop your horse in different places where he can explore. It can also be stopping just to smell the dung of other horses, although you have to be sure that there are no infectious diseases going around.

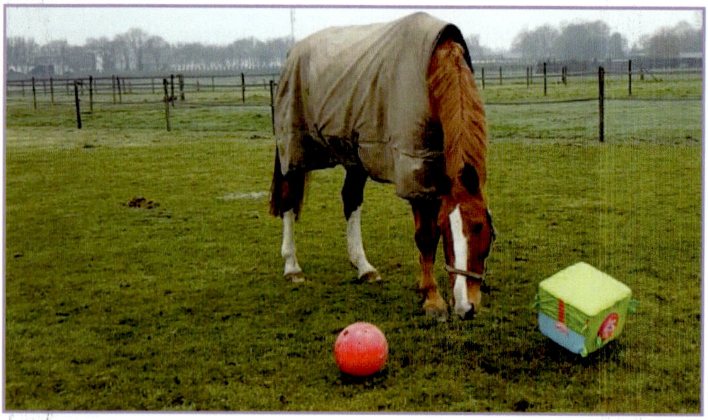

Fig. 5.14 An example of an enriched environment.

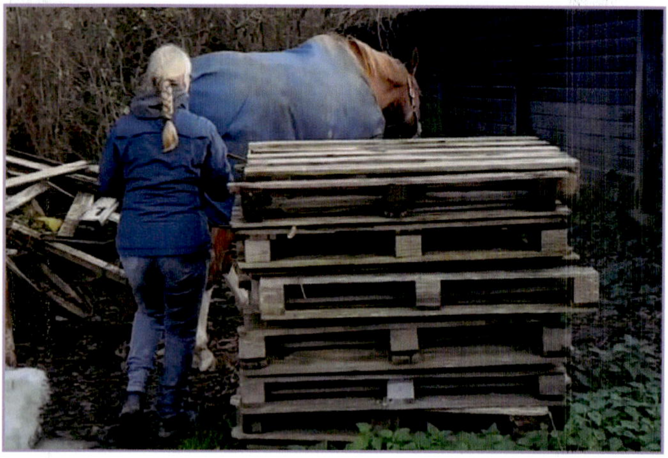

Fig. 5.15 An example of a real-life enriched environment.

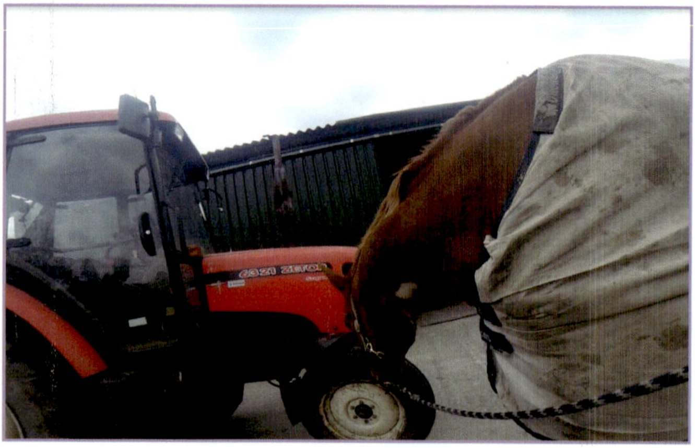

Fig. 5.16 I see if Vosje wants to examine a tractor standing in the yard. Notice the rope is slack – I am standing behind Vosje. He decides the pace of discovery.

TRACKING GAMES

Horses have an extraordinarily good sense of smell. Although it is hard to pinpoint exactly how good, especially in comparison to other mammals, researchers have tried. For instance, Ramesh Padodara, Laurie Issel-Tarver, Jasper Rine and Yoshihito Niimura *et al* compared the intact functional olfactory receptor genes of various mammals including horses, dogs and humans. The size of the olfactory bulb and nasal epithelium were also studied. The assumption is that the better the olfactory capability of an animal is, the more intact functional olfactory receptor genes the animal has and the bigger its olfactory bulb. If you combine the results of the above mentioned researchers with the numbers in the book *Neuroscience* by Purves *et al*, *The Mind of the Horse* by Michel-Antoine Leblanc and the study by Boniface M. Kavoi and Hassanali Jameela, you will find that the olfactory capabilities of a horse are placed slightly below that of dogs but much better than that of a human. Riders are often aware of their horse's sense of smell if he becomes tense after catching a scent, but horse's sense of smell is not often used as an additional tool. This is unfortunate, because tracking can bring many advantages:

- By letting the horse experience the world by smelling, he gets to know it better, making him less fearful of it and better able to socialise.
- It makes the horse more independent and gives him confidence. With his nose, he can accomplish things we cannot.
- It appeals to the horse's natural abilities. This produces dopamines, which make the horse feel better.[2]
- The more you track, the more motivated the horse becomes. This is not just because of the reward, but because of the activity itself.[2]
- It is mentally challenging and tiring.
- It calms.
- It serves very well as an exercise if the horse needs to be distracted.
- It is a good exercise if horses are not allowed or able to move much.
- It is a fun exercise for both horse and handler, and it promotes team spirit.

There are many advantages to using a horse's tracking abilities. By stimulating senses such as smell, sight, and hearing, you can give your horse's mental stimulation a boost. This is especially useful because in training programmes there is often an imbalance between the many physical exercises a horse has to do and the minimal mental ones. The horses I have done tracking exercises with came to enjoy them very much. The biggest challenge is to sufficiently stimulate the horse in the first place for him to participate, especially if he can also choose to eat instead. Therefore, in tracking it helps if the horse is not initially hungry. However, once the horse gets the hang of these exercises, he is in. I learned the games listed below during Turid Rugaas's International Dog Trainer School and Anne Lill Kvam's Nosework Education programme. These exercises were originally meant for dogs, but they are also suitable for horses. Tracking games you can do include:

- **Treat search.** Finding scattered pieces of food on different surfaces. Vary the colours and size to make it easier or more difficult.

- **Food track.** Following a food track, in which the distance between bits of food increases as the exercise becomes more difficult.
- **Scent discrimination (Fig. 5.17).** Picking the correct herbs from a collection of herbs.
- **Man trailing (Fig. 5.18).** Finding the owner or an animal by following their trail.
- **Scent garden.** Spreading scents over a part of the paddock is also very interesting and stimulating for a horse.
- **Searching for a towel.** You vary the places where you hide the towel from easy (in a corner of the paddock, behind a tuft of grass) to difficult (over a tree branch).
- **Smelling reality.** Giving your horse a chance to sniff around in his environment. The exercises can be made more difficult by varying the ground on which you do them.

When tracking, it is important to read your horse's body language. This enables you to know when to call breaks. Tracking is tiring. Do short sessions with ample breaks in between.

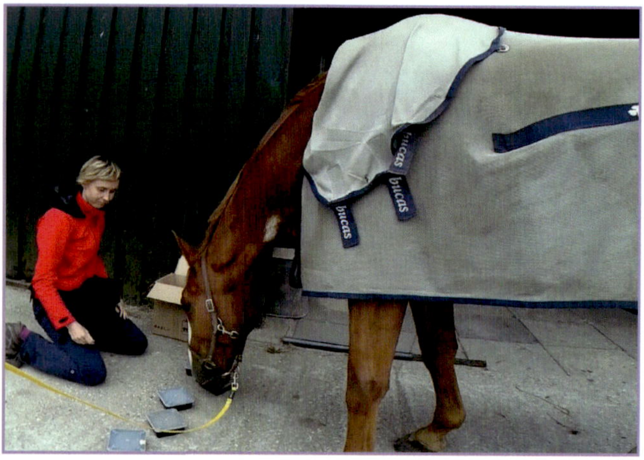

Fig. 5.17 Els is doing scent discrimination. Vosje indicates the herb we were looking for: dill. Every container has one herb in it. The lids have holes in them so the horse can smell the herbs.

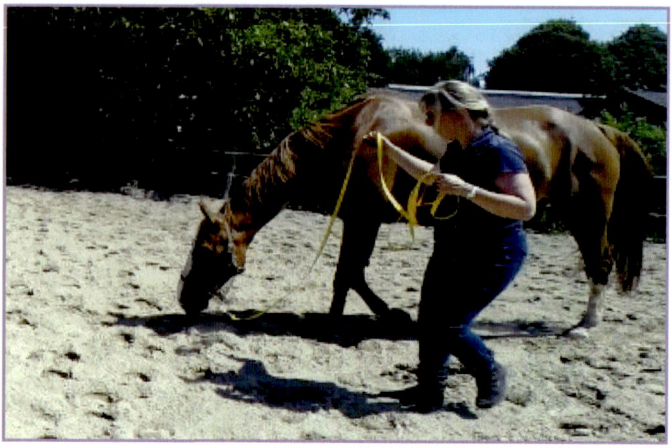

Fig. 5.18 Human trailing. Vosje is looking for Els by following her scent trail.

GAMES THAT STIMULATE THE SENSES

Described below are some games that stimulate the sense of smell, but also other senses:

- **Tasty waters.** Offering buckets of water to which you have added a few drops of flavouring, such as apple juice, tea, or tomato juice.
- **Ball or bottle box.** Place lots of balls or lidless bottles in a large box. The horse can rummage around in the box, trying to extract an apple or some other treat.
- **Dry or wet towel game.** You hide an apple under a dry or wet towel. The horse can get the (piece of) apple by removing the towel. You can make this more difficult by folding the towel a number of times.
- **Crate stacking game.** You put an apple inside a light grocery crate. The horse can take it out. Then you put another apple in, but place another empty crate on top of the first one. The horse starts by moving the top crate slightly, but eventually he has to topple the crate over completely to get to the apple. You can build the crate tower even higher and vary the crate in which you place the treat. You can also play the game on different surfaces. In my experience, horses are less startled by loud noises if they know they have caused them themselves, but you can start on a soft surface and work towards a hard one.
- **Apples on a string.** Core apples, string them on a rope (in slices if need be), and let the horse eat them off the rope. You can hang the rope between poles or tie it to a tree branch.
- **Bread beams.** Place old, hardened bread between beams lying on the ground. The horse needs to move the beams aside a bit to get to the bread.

In all games safety first is the most important issue. No game should hurt or create fear. It is only fun if the horse enjoys the game and wants to participate in it. If the game is too difficult, make it easier. The goal is always that the horse should be able to solve any problem, even if it takes him multiple sessions to do so. Remember that most horses are not used to taking a personal initiative, especially with the owner present. Sometimes it takes them a while to discover that playing is fun. So this sometimes has to be actively tapped into.

5.11 SUMMARY: TIPS

- It is a basic responsibility to care for every horse in such a way that he is heathy, pain free, neither hungry nor thirsty, that he has shelter, that he can go out to pasture for at least a couple of hours every day, and that he is in contact with other horses who make a good match for him. For his emotional wellbeing, it is also important that a horse is allowed to make choices, enabling him to better understand and control the world around him.
- Communication ladders are intended as assessment tools to help you recognise and, to a certain extent, predict your horse's behaviour. It is challenging to look at signals from a horse who is experiencing shifting internal motivations. This is reflected in a pendular pattern on the communication ladder.
- Sound planning is indispensable when dealing with horses. You should avoid negative experiences and fear emotions, focus on the horse's signals and try to have him associate positive, relaxed emotions with experiences.
- Create many opportunities for relaxation. Do not punish the horse. Do not leave your horse alone and use hand signals.
- Use calming signals (such as splitting, curving, turning your side or back, doing a head turn or shoulder turn, or standing still) yourself.
- Respond to the communication signals the horse is giving, possibly abandoning your own wishes.
- Empower your horse: make him more independent and able to handle himself. This will improve his cognition and memory and will decrease his fear and aggression responses as well as his overreactions. You do this by reducing your own control, by giving the horse freedom to choose within a safe space.
- Other tools are: creating enriched environments, having your horse do tracking, and playing games with him.

5.12 REFERENCES

1 Panksepp J (2015) *The Science of Emotions*. Lecture at Kamerik, The Netherlands.
2 Panksepp J, Biven L (2012) *The Archaeology of Mind: Neuroevolutionary Origins of Human Emotions*. W.W. Norton & Company, New York, pp. 95–105.
3 National Scientific Council on the Developing Child (2014) *Excessive Stress Disrupts the Architecture of the Developing Brain: Working Paper 3*. Updated Edition. http://developingchild.harvard.edu/resources/wp3/
4 Swaab D (2010) *Wij zijn ons brein. Van baarmoeder tot alzheimer*. Olympus, Amsterdam, p. 41.
5 Panksepp J, Biven L (2012) *The Archaeology of Mind: Neuroevolutionary Origins of Human Emotions*. W.W. Norton & Company, New York, p. 373.
6 Panksepp J, Biven L (2012) *The Archaeology of Mind: Neuroevolutionary Origins of Human Emotions*. W.W. Norton & Company, New York, p. 106.
7 Neugebauer GM, Neugebauer JK (2011) *Het gedrag van paarden beter begrijpen.* Eugen Ulmer KG, Stuttgart, p. 26.

Appendices

A1 EYES (Figs A1.1–A1.8)

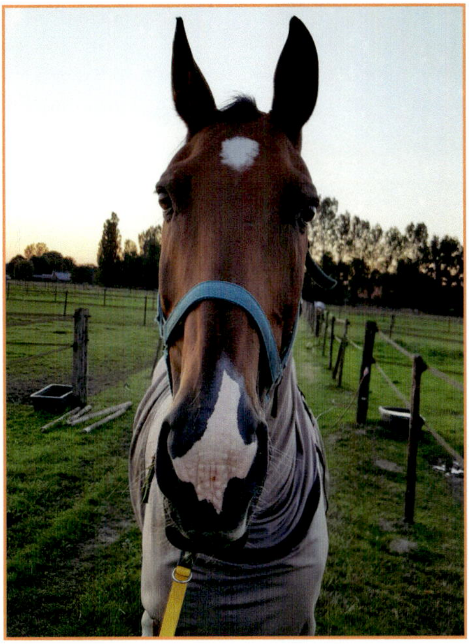

Fig. A1.1 Looking straight ahead.

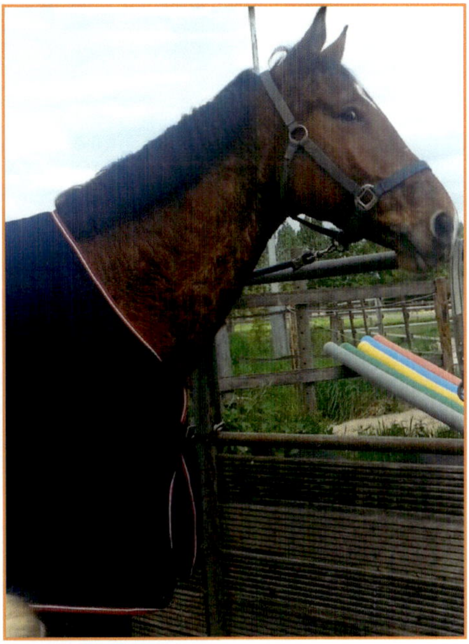

Fig. A1.2 Looking to the side without doing a head turn.

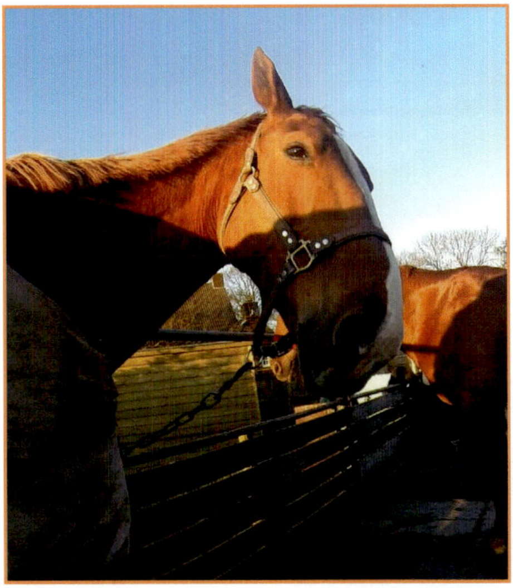

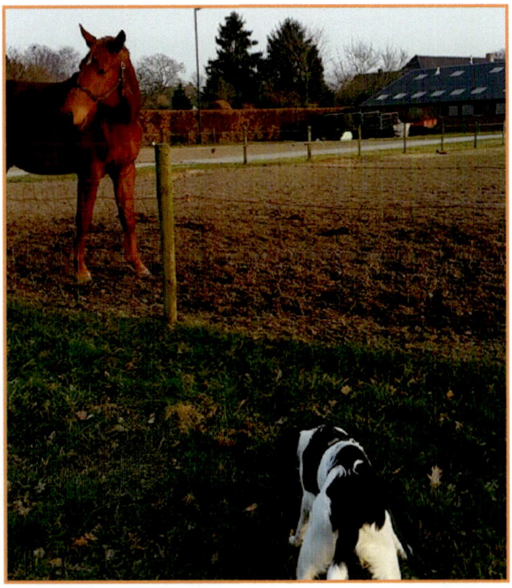

Figs A1.3, A1.4 Looking by turning the head.

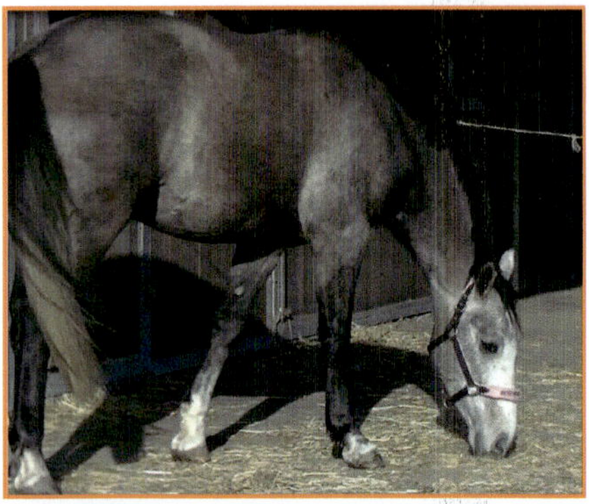

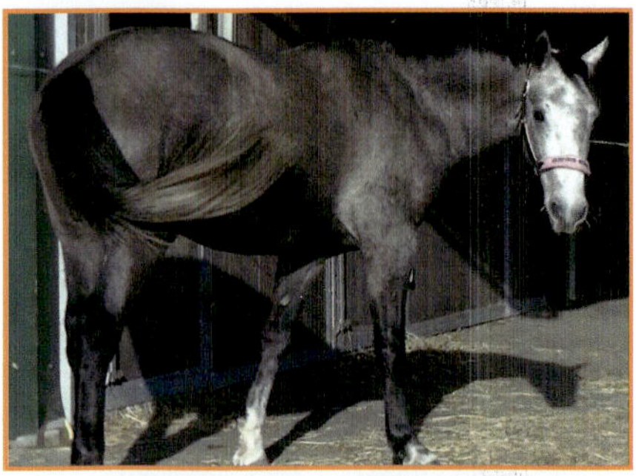

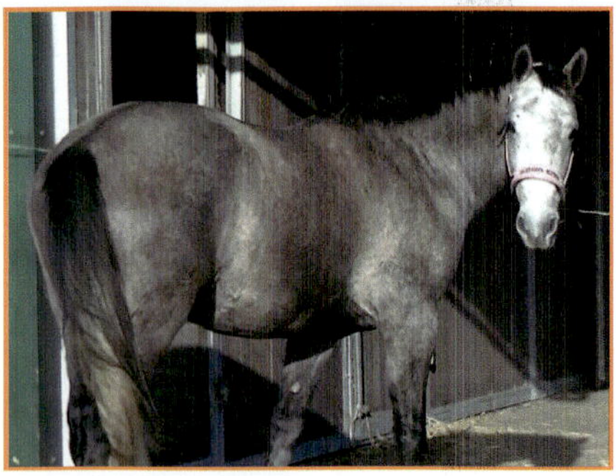

Figs A1.5–A1.7 A combination.

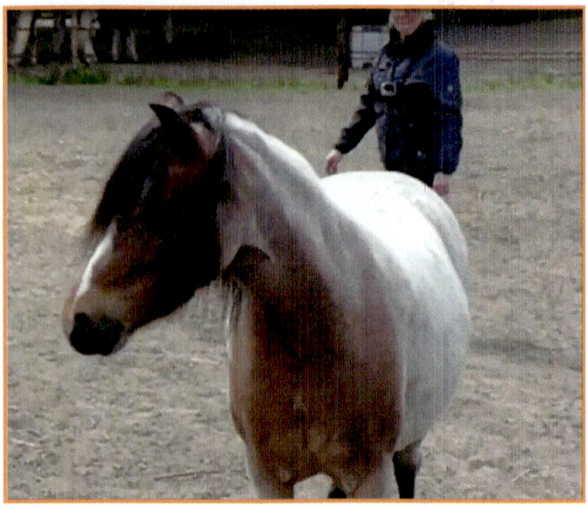

Fig. A1.8 Looking back.

A2 EARS

If you look at how the ears behave, you will see that they are very flexible. They can move synchronously (both at the same time) or they can move independently from one another. They can make a ninety-degree turn and catch sounds that are coming from the front, from the side, or from the back. When confronted with a stimulus, ears respectively turn towards the place on which the attention is focused (**Fig. A2.1**) or the place from which the sound is coming. They can demonstrate this through various ear positions and the degree to which the ear positions change (**Figs A2.2–A2.6**). The better the horse is able to handle his environment, the more calmly his ears move.

Both ears forwards

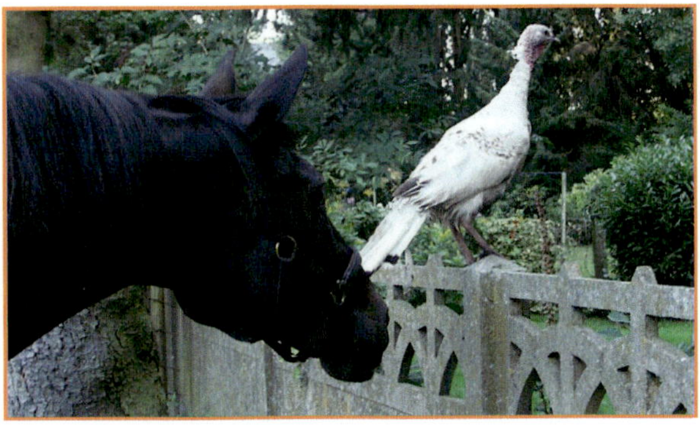

Fig. A2.1 Pointing to where the attention is focused.

One ear turned sideways or back

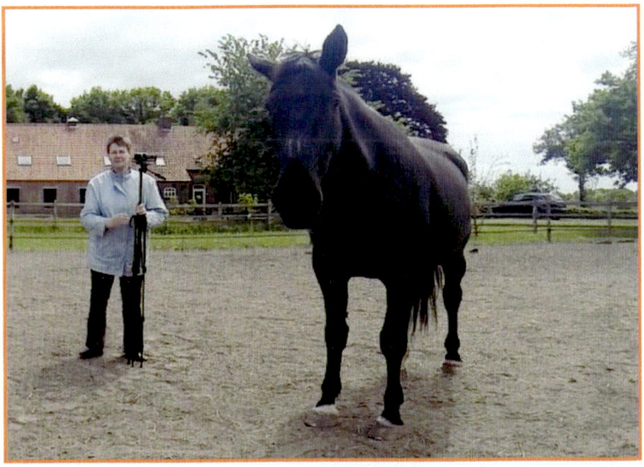

Fig. A2.2 Focusing on a particular stimulus or several stimuli. Pearl is being filmed by Ristin and me. By her ears you can tell where we are standing. One of Pearl's ears points to Ristin. I am standing in front of Pearl. Her other ear points to me.

Both ears turned back

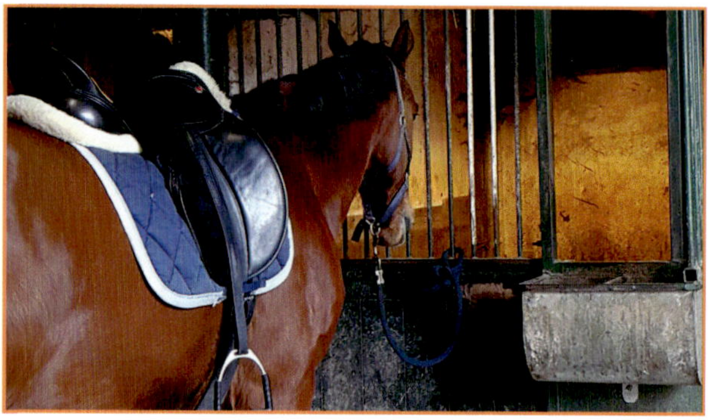

Fig. A2.3 When catching a sound coming from behind.

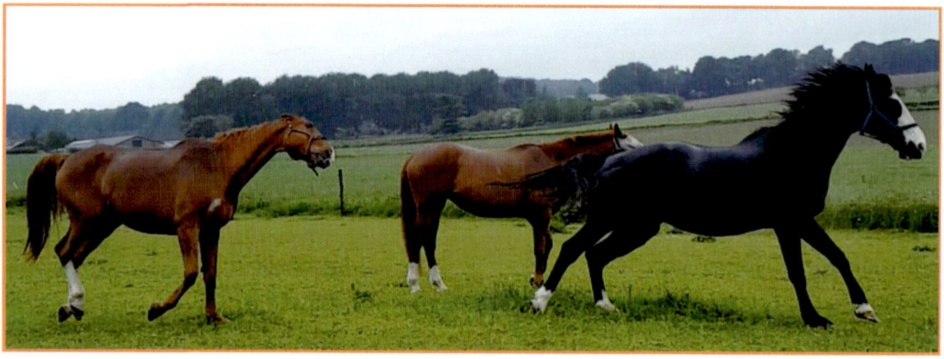

Fig. A2.4 When using distance increasing signals, for example.

Both ears turned sideways

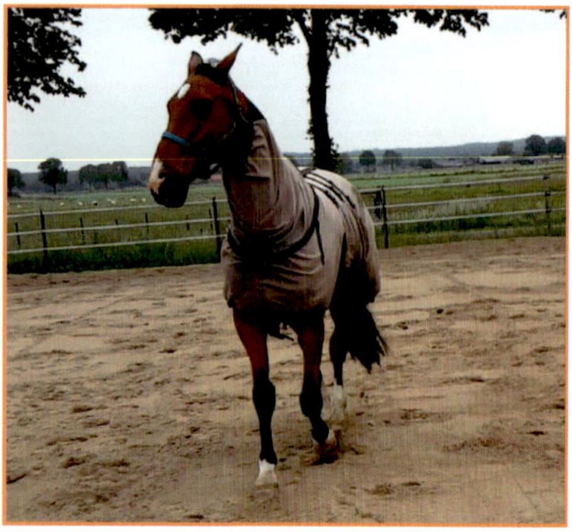

Fig. A2.5 In a situation of weak and strong flight behaviour.

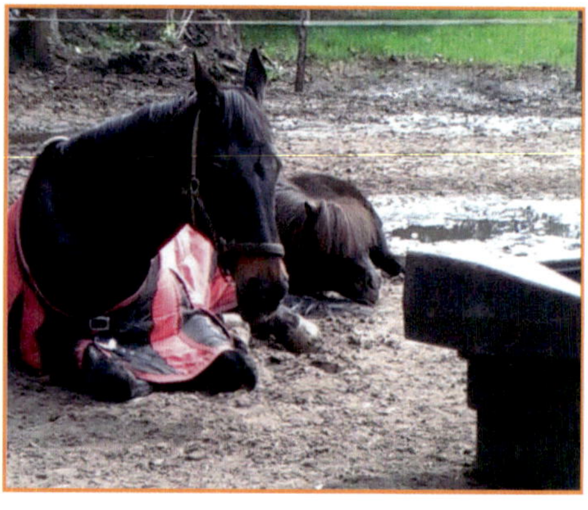

Fig. A2.6 This occurs when the horse is trying to catch sounds from both sides, when he is asleep or falling asleep, when he is in pain, or in a situation of learned helplessness and depression.

Bibliography (personal favourites)

Bekoff M (2008) *The Emotional Lives of Animals*. New World Library, Novato.

Gazzano A, Mariti C, Papi F, Falaschi C, Forti S (2010) Are domestic dogs able to calm conspecifics by visual communication? *J Vet Behav* **5(1)**.

De Giorgio F, Schoorl J (2014) *The Cognitive Horse: An Inspiring Journey Towards a New Co-existence.* Learning Animals, Nistelrode.

Kainer RA, McCracken TO (1998) *Horse Anatomy: A Coloring Atlas, Second Edition.* Alpine Publications, Crawford.

Konturek PC, Brzozowski T, Konturek SJ (2011) Stress and the gut: pathophysiology, clinical consequences, diagnostic approach and treatment options. *J Physiol Pharmacol* **62(6):**591–599.

Kvam A-L (2012) *The Canine Kingdom of Scent.* Dogwise Publishing, Wenatchee.

Mariti C, Falaschi C, Zilocchi M, Carlone B, Gazano A (2014) Analysis of calming signals in domestic dogs; Are they signals and are they calming? *J Vet Behav* **9(6)**.

Mariti C, Papi F, Ducci M, Sighieri C, Martelli F (2010) Domestic dogs display calming signals more frequently towards unfamiliar rather than familiar dogs. *J Vet Behav* **5(1)**.

McBane S (2012) *Horse Senses.* Manson Publishing Ltd, London.

McDonnel S (2003) *A Practical Field Guide to Horse Behaviour: The Equid Ethogram*. The Blood-Horse, Lexington.

McEwen BS (2004) Protection and damage from acute and chronic stress. Allostasis and allostatic overload and relevance to the pathophysiology of psychiatric disorders. *Ann N Y Acad Sci* **1032:**1–7.

McEwen BS (2008) Central effects of stress hormones in health and disease: understanding the protective and damaging effects of stress and stress mediators. *Europ J Pharmacol* **583(2–3):**174–185.

McGreevy P, McLean A (2010) *Equitation Science.* Wiley-Blackwell, Hoboken.

Mönki J, Hewetson M, Virtala AM (2016) Risk factors for equine gastric glandular disease: a case-control study in finnish referral hospital population. *J Vet Intern Med,* **30(4)**:1270–1275. https://www.researchgate.net/publication/305692704_Risk_Factors_for_Equine_Gastric_Glandular_Disease_A_Case-Control_Study_in_a_Finnish_Referral_Hospital_Population

National Scientific Council on the Developing Child (2005/2014) Excessive Stress Disrupts the Architecture of the Developing Brain: working paper 3. Updated Edition. http://developingchild.harvard.edu/resources/wp3/

Neugebauer GM, Neugebauer JK (2011) *Het gedrag van paarden beter begrijpen.* Eugen Ulmer KG, Stuttgart, p. 26.

Panksepp J, Biven L (2012) *The Archaeology of Mind: Neuroevolutionary Origins of Human Emotions.* W.W. Norton & Company, New York.

Robertson J (2010) *The Complete Dog Massage Manual*. Hubble & Hattie, Poundbury.

Robertson J, Mead A (2013) *Physical Therapy and Massage of the Dog.* Manson Publishing, London.

Rugaas T (2002) *Kalmerende Signalen, wat u en uw hond elkaar vertellen.* Yggdrasil.

Rugaas T (2008) *Blafgedraf van honden, wat betekent het en hoe kun je ermee omgaan.* Yggdrasil.

Seligman ME, Maier SF (1967) Failure to escape traumatic shock. *J Exper Psychol* **74(1):**1–9.

Society for Endocrinology (2015) What is anti-diuretic hormone? http://www.yourhormones.info/hormones/antidiuretic_hormone.aspx

Spiers W, Dydon O (2008) *How to Handle Living With Your Dog.* Short Stack Publishing, Stratford Upon Avon.

Swaab D (2010) *Wij zijn ons brein, van baarmoeder tot Alzheimer.* Olympus, Amsterdam, p. 41.

Sykes BW, Hewetson M, Hepburn RJ, Luthersson N, Tamzali Y, European College of Equine Internal Medicine Consensus Statement – Equine Gastric Ulcer Syndrome in Adult Horses. https://www.ncbi.nlm.nih.gov/pmc/articles/PMC4858038/

VanFleet R (2012) *The Human Half of Dog Training.* Dogwise Publishing, Wenatchee.

VanFleet R, Faa-Thompson T (2017) *Animal Assisted Play Therapy.* Professional Resource Press, Sarasota.

de Waal F (2016) *Zijn we slim genoeg om te weten hoe slim dieren zijn? (Are we smart enough to know how smart animals are?).* Atlas contact, Amsterdam.

Waran N (ed) (2003) *The Welfare of Horses.* Kluwer Academic Publishers, Berlin.

Zo Werkt Het Lichaam (How it Works Body): de fysiologie, anatomie en pathologie van het menselijk lichaam (Physiology, Pathology, and Anatomy of the Human Body), Zenuwstelsel: parasympatisch en sympathisch zenuwstelsel (Nervous system: parasympathetic and sympathetic nervous system) http://www.zowerkthetlichaam.nl/3068/zenuwstelsel-parasympatisch-en-sympatisch-zenuwstelsel/

Index